Advancing Responsible Adolescent Development

Series Editor

Roger J.R. Levesque
Indiana University, Bloomington, IN, U.S.A.

For further volumes:
http://www.springer.com/series/7284

H. Harrington Cleveland · Kitty S. Harris · Richard P. Wiebe

Editors

Substance Abuse Recovery in College

Community Supported Abstinence

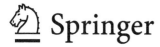 Springer

Editors
H. Harrington Cleveland
Department of Human Development &
  Family Studies
Pennsylvania State University
University Park PA 16802
USA
hhc10@psu.edu

Kitty S. Harris
Texas Tech University
Center for the Study of Addiction
  and Recovery
Lubbock TX 79409
Box 41162
USA
kitty.s.harris@ttu.edu

Richard P. Wiebe
Department of Behavioral Sciences
Fitchburg State College
160 Pearl Street
Fitchburg MA 01420
USA
rwiebe@fsc.edu

ISBN 978-1-4419-1766-9   e-ISBN 978-1-4419-1767-6
DOI 10.1007/978-1-4419-1767-6
Springer New York Dordrecht Heidelberg London

Library of Congress Control Number: 2010920306

Printed on acid-free paper

Springer is part of Springer Science+Business Media (www.springer.com)

Preface

More than 80% of college students are drinking. More than a third do drugs. For students struggling with substance abuse, temptations on campus—and stressors that can derail abstinence—run high. In response, several colleges and universities offer effective support in the form of recovery communities, which are more appropriate to campus settings and young adult development than traditional 12-step groups alone.

Substance Abuse Recovery in College explains in authoritative detail what collegiate recovery communities are, the types of services they provide, and their role in the context of campus life, with extended examples from Texas Tech University's influential CSAR (Center for the Study of Addiction and Recovery) program. Using data from both conventional surveys and end-of-day daily Palm Pilot assessments as well as focus groups, the book examines community members' experiences. In addition, the importance of a positive relationship between the recovery community and the school administration is emphasized.

Topics covered include:

- The growing need for recovery services at colleges.
- How recovery communities support abstinence and relapse prevention.
- Who are community members and their addiction and treatment histories.
- Daily lives of young adults in a collegiate recovery community.
- Challenges and opportunities in establishing recovery communities on campus.
- Building abstinence support into an academic curriculum.

This volume offers clear insights and up-close perspectives of importance to developmental and clinical child psychologists, social workers, higher education policymakers, and related professionals in human development, family studies, student services, college health care, and community services.

University Park, Pennsylvania   H. Harrington Cleveland
Lubbock, Texas   Kitty S. Harris
Fitchburg, Massachusetts   Richard P. Wiebe

Acknowledgments

The editors and authors of this volume acknowledge the support of the College of Human Sciences at Texas Tech University, which provided funding for much of the research presented herein. Specifically, we would like to thank Dean Linda Hoover, who helped Dr. Cleveland acquire the Palm Pilots used to collect the data used for Chapter 6. We wish to thank Dr. Evelyn Moser for her reading and commenting on early drafts of the chapters. In addition, it should be noted that the data presented in Chapter 4 includes research that has been published in the *Journal of Substance Abuse Treatment*. The full cite to the original research article is Cleveland, H. H., Harris, K. S., Baker, A., Herbert, R., & Dean, L. R. (2007). Characteristics of a Collegiate Recovery Community: Safe Haven in an Abstinence Hostile Collegiate Environment. *Journal of Substance Abuse Treatment, 33*, 13– 23. The *Journal of Substance Abuse Treatment* has approved the republishing of these data. It should also be acknowledged that Chapter 8, Building Support for Recovery into an Academic Curriculum: Student Reflections on the Value of Staff Run Seminars, is the result of a Program Evaluation course facilitated by the second author, Miriam Mulsow, Ph.D. We respectfully thank Diane Oliver, Ph.D., who assisted in the evaluation. We also thank students of the class listed above whose hard work and dedication contributed to the evaluation: Gail Bentley, Augustina Brooks, Holly Follmer, Janis Henderson, Greg Johnston, and Yingli Li.

Contents

Contributors

Amanda Baker Texas Tech University, Lubbock, TX, USA,
amanda.k.baker@ttu.edu

Ann M. Casiraghi Texas Tech University, Lubbock, TX, USA,
anne.m.casiraghi@ttu.edu

H. Harrington Cleveland The Pennsylvania State University, University Park,
PA, USA, cleveland@psu.edu

Lukas R. Dean The William Paterson University, Wayne, NJ, USA,
deanl1@wpunj.edu

Allison Groenendyk The Pennsylvania State University, University Park,
PA, USA, allison.groenendyk@gmail.com

Kitty S. Harris Texas Tech University, Lubbock, TX, USA, kitty.s.harris@ttu.edu

Miriam Mulsow Texas Tech University, Lubbock, TX, USA,
miriam.mulsow@ttu.edu

Matthew Russell Texas Tech University, Lubbock TX, USA,
matthew.russell@ttu.edu

Richard P. Wiebe Fitchburg State College, Fitchburg, MA, USA, rwiebe@fsc.edu

Jacquelyn D. Wiersma The Pennsylvania State University, University Park,
PA, USA, jdw22@psu.edu

Chapter 1
The Need for College Recovery Services

Richard P. Wiebe, H. Harrington Cleveland, and Kitty S. Harris

> *You have four years to be irresponsible here. Relax. Work is for*
> *people with jobs. You'll never remember class time, but you'll*
> *remember time you wasted hanging out with your friends. So,*
> *stay out late. Go out on a Tuesday with your friends when you*
> *have a paper due Wednesday. Spend money you don't have.*
> *Drink 'til sunrise. The work never ends, but college does.*
> –Tom Petty
> *College is the best time of your life. When else are your parents*
> *going to spend several thousand dollars a year just for you to go*
> *to a strange town and get drunk every night?*
> –David Wood

For too many college students, college represents the last bastion of adolescent irresponsibility. On most college campuses, drugs and alcohol are widely available, and students are loudly exhorted by peers and other social and cultural influences to drink and use drugs, with excessive substance use often seen as a rite of passage (National Center on Addiction and Substance Abuse at Columbia University [CASA], 2007). This environment may be appealing to the minds of some college students. However, for young adults in recovery from drug or alcohol addiction, it is difficult to imagine, let alone find, a setting more hostile to maintaining abstinence than a college campus (Cleveland, Harris, Baker, Herbert, & Dean, 2007).

America's campuses are in the midst of a substance use epidemic that shows no sign of abating. A nationally representative survey by CASA revealed that while the proportion of college students who drank decreased from 70 to 68% between 1993 and 2005 (a statistically insignificant decline) and the number who binge drank at least once a week remained at 40%, rates of frequent drinking, frequent binge drinking, and drinking to get drunk among college students increased during the same period by 25, 16, and 21%, respectively (CASA, 2007; see also Dowdall & Wechsler, 2002). These drinking behaviors track the increasing cultural importance of drinking to the college experience (Schulenberg & Maggs, 2002). Together, the

R.P. Wiebe (✉)
Fitchburg State College, Fitchburg, MA, USA
e-mail: rwiebe@fsc.edu

H.H. Cleveland et al. (eds.), *Substance Abuse Recovery in College*, Advancing
Responsible Adolescent Development, DOI 10.1007/978-1-4419-1767-6_1,
© Springer Science+Business Media, LLC 2010

1

behavioral prevalence and cultural centrality of drinking have created a culture that affects everyone exposed to it (Presley, Meilman, & Leichliter, 2002). Students who come to college drinking, drink more. And many non-drinkers or moderate drinkers are induced to take up heavy drinking (Wechsler & Weuthrich, 2002).

These behaviors are dangerous for everyone. Among college students aged 18–24, alcohol-related unintentional injury deaths increased from nearly 1,600 to more than 1,700 (increase of 6% per college population) between 1998 and 2001. During the same period, the proportion of students who reported driving under the influence of alcohol rose from 26.5%, or 2.3 million, to 31.4%, or 2.8 million (Hingson, Heeren, Winter, & Wechsler, 2005).

This atmosphere of collegiate drinking reflects trends among American youth generally. For example, the 2007 Youth Risk Behavior Survey found that among high school students, during the past 30 days, 45% drank some amount of alcohol, 26% engaged in binge drinking, 11% drove after drinking alcohol, and 29% rode with a driver who had been drinking alcohol (Eaton et al., 2008). And the Substance Abuse and Mental Health Services Administration (SAMHSA) reported that among Americans aged 12–17, 5.8% had begun to use illicit drugs and 10.7% had begun to use alcohol during 2007 (SAMHSA, 2008).

Of course, college students do more than just drink. Illicit drug use among students increased even more than serious drinking during the period covered by the CASA survey. Daily marijuana use more than doubled, illegal hard drug use went up 52%, and abuse of prescription drugs increased by 93% for stimulants such as Ritalin, 225% for sedatives such as Nembutal, 343% for synthetic opiates such as OxyContin, and 450% for tranquilizers such as Xanex (CASA, 2007). Altogether, each month, almost half (49.4%) of all full-time college students aged 18–22 either binge drink, abuse prescription or illegal drugs, or both, and about 22.9% of those students meet diagnostic criteria for substance abuse or dependence, almost triple the rate of the general population (8.5%).

Barriers to Maintaining Recovery

While it has been widely recognized that the college drinking environment threatens the health and well-being of college students generally, there has been little focus on how it affects students who enter college already struggling with addictions to alcohol and other drugs. The pool of these potential student addicts is large; for example, the Substance Abuse and Mental Health Services and Administration reported for the year 2003 that 1,500,000 individuals between the ages of 12 and 17 either regularly abused alcohol or were alcohol dependent (SAMHSA, 2007). Not surprisingly, the number of adolescents entering treatment has increased more than those from other age groups, rising 65% in the decade ending in 2003 compared to 23% for the population as a whole (SAMHSA). It is hard to imagine individuals who are more threatened by an alcohol-centered social context than those who are trying to maintain recoveries from addictions.

Recovery is a day-to-day process, not a "cure" for abuse or addiction (Humphries, 2004; see Maruna, 2001), and it requires a lifelong commitment to recognizing the need for and seeking external help when necessary (Vaillant, 2005). For young men and women in recovery, partaking in any alcohol or drug use could trigger life-threatening sequelae of abuse. Faced with the prospect of risking their hard-won abstinence, many in recovery from substance abuse and addiction consider going to college, whether for the first time or as returning students, an unacceptable risk. Campus social environments present myriad challenges and difficulties for these vulnerable young men and women. They may have difficulty resisting social pressures toward group conformity in what appears to be an alcohol-saturated environment (Perkins, 2002). They may feel shut out of college social life, even the substance-free activities, where discussions often turn to recent or future events involving drug and alcohol use. They may experience stress from the constant bombardment of alcohol ads in and around the campus environment.

Compounding these difficulties, recovering students may not be able to find or build the social networks they need to support their abstinence lifestyle. On one hand, their "normal" nonrecovery college peers will have no idea how dangerous any use of substances at all can be for them. On the other hand, conventional recovery support groups, on which individuals seeking recovery support would normally rely, are largely composed of older adults. The differences in current age and life context, as well as differences in how addictions affected their lives because of their being adolescents rather than adults during the period of their active addictions, can interfere with young adults finding support, identification, and a sense of commonality within the fellowships offered by conventional mutual help support groups (Harrison & Hoffman, 1987). The lack of perceived support by "normal" peers in a collegiate environment and the potential difficulty of identifying with other members of recovery support groups can make staying clean and sober seem virtually impossible in a college environment.

The problems faced by recovering college students stem not only from the college environment, with its emphasis on getting wasted and lack of social support for abstinence, but from the developmental challenges that can come with their histories of addictive adolescent substance use. The teen years are the time of life when both individual (Erikson, 1968) and social (Barber, Eccles, & Stone, 2001) identities are formed. The direct and indirect effects of substance abuse during these formative years can interfere with healthy development, leaving recovering college students ill-prepared to deal with the abstinence-hostile environment of college. Further, late adolescence and early adulthood are when the risk of all behaviors evincing low self-control, including but not limited to substance use, is at their peak and low self-control increases the risk of falling prey to antisocial peer influences, such as the pressure to drink and use drugs (Gottfredson & Hirschi, 1990).

It is admittedly difficult for colleges to make a wholesale change in the drinking culture that persists on college campuses (CASA, 2007). But the seeming intractability of the larger culture of alcohol use and abuse on college campuses is not a reason to ignore the needs of the growing numbers of young adults in recovery from alcohol and other drugs. Colleges can play an active role in protecting the abstinence of those in substance abuse recovery. In doing so, colleges can not only provide access to education for those who are challenged by addictions, but also demonstrate to all their students that college life is not synonymous with substance abuse. Colleges and universities can do this by establishing collegiate recovery communities. Without these communities, it will be difficult for the growing numbers of young men and women in recovery to complete their educations, without which they will be less able to build successful and stable careers.

By developing recovery communities, colleges and universities can provide safe havens from the drinking and drug abuse that permeate college life. This book presents the story of the Collegiate Recovery Community at Texas Tech University (TTU), which is one of the oldest and largest collegiate recovery communities in the United States. In doing so, it provides details on the need for these communities, the theoretical foundations of the program that supports the community, who the members of the community are, what daily life is like in the community, the extent of social network protection provided by community membership, how the community is linked to the program that supports it via academic seminars, and how the TTU program is assisting other colleges and universities build their own collegiate recovery communities, with the support of Center for Substance Abuse and Treatment of the US Department of Health and Human Services and the US Department of Education.

Overview of This Book

Why aren't 12-step programs adequate for the task of helping college students maintain recovery, and what does a college recovery community have that a traditional 12-step program doesn't? Chapter 2 answers these questions, while noting that 12-step programs constitute an important element of a successful collegiate recovery community. The authors detail the growth in the population served by collegiate recovery communities and discuss the development of college recovery communities across the country in general and at the largest of these communities in particular. They review the different models for collegiate recovery communities, with an emphasis on contrasting the Rutgers model, widely considered the first significant collegiate recovery community (Rutgers University Health Services, 2001), with the model developed at the Center for the Study of Addiction and Recovery (CSAR) at TTU, which embodies many of the principles elucidated by Salzer (2002).

Chapter 3 examines the unique challenges that addictive substance use can present to the developmental tasks of adolescence through the lens of Erik Erikson's pioneering work in lifespan developmental psychology. The authors discuss how substance use can derail normal adolescent identity development, leaving the teenaged addict uniquely unprepared to face the stressors inherent in the American college experience. And they discuss how different components of the Collegiate Recovery Community (CRC) run by the CSAR address the challenge of identity formation among young addicts.

Any recovery program should account for and be understood in regard to the unique characteristics and needs of the individuals it serves. Chapter 4 introduces us to the members of the CRC at TTU. We learn that they are a group of motivated and able young men and women who work hard at recovery. We also learn that their substance use histories are serious, and their successes in recovery and academic work are correspondingly impressive.

With only a 4% relapse rate per semester, the members of the CRC generally succeed in their recoveries. Chapter 5 details the results of a study assessing the urges to use substances faced by CRC members and the tactics they use to deal with these urges. The most important of these tactics involve social support rather than physical interventions such as medications. The material in Chapter 5 profoundly illustrates the dictum that recovery is a process, and the addict must remain ever vigilant, never assuming that the urge to use will ever simply disappear.

As Chapter 5 establishes the importance of social support for maintaining recovery, the question arises: Exactly what kind of social support to CRC members receive? Using daily diary data drawn from over 50 members of the CRC, Chapter 6 presents a detailed study of exactly how and with whom CRC members spend their time. Within the largest recovery community of its type, CRC members have numerous potential sources of abstinent-specific friendships; in a smaller community, members might feel constrained by the limited number of peers who really "get it." As this chapter illustrates, by supporting the CRC community the CSAR provides a large number of varied settings that are safe for recovering students and that help them maintain their recovery. An important finding of Chapter 6 is that community members venture often into the wider university community, going to football games, parties, bars, and other social settings where alcohol at least is widely available and its use encouraged, but are still able to maintain their recoveries using the tactics described in Chapter 5. Moreover, this chapter demonstrates that it is the community supported by the CSAR program, rather than the program itself, that provides the majority of both the social support necessary for abstinence and the social experiences necessary for individual development of community members as detailed by Chapter 3. Finally, this chapter also documents the substantially variability in the daily social experiences, including those experiences that would seem to challenge recovery of community members. Thus, like all prevention efforts, the CSAR program does not work in the same way for everyone.

While Chapter 6 provides a day-to-day feel of how and where CRC members spend their time, Chapter 7 takes a more conventional approach to quantifying social network support and risk. Prior research has demonstrated that social network support, specifically the number of abstinent social network members versus the number of substance-using social network members, is a primary factor in predicting continued abstinence (Beattie & Longabaugh, 1999; Zywiak, Longabaugh, & Wirtz, 2002). Chapter 7 gives information on the extent to which community members' social networks are stocked with abstainers. By using data derived from a version of an established social network measure, the Inventory of Important People and Activities (IPA; Zywiak et al., 2002) tailored for the recovery status of CRC members, this chapter demonstrates the effectiveness of the CSAR program in providing a community that literally saturates its members with social support for abstinence, while providing them with the opportunities for normative social interactions they require to develop healthy identities that integrate a strong sense of personal and social selves necessary for both current sobriety and sustained recovery.

Together with Chapter 5, Chapter 7 illustrates the importance of social support delivered by peers and other individuals who are intimately familiar with the problems faced by the recovering addict. This kind of social support is called "abstinence-specific."

One of the central components of the CSAR program is the Seminar for Recovering Students (Seminar), a course in which each CRC member is required to register each semester. Chapter 8 examines the role of Seminar in the recovery of CRC members, and provides a detailed overview of various types of social support and the components of the CSAR program designed to deliver them. This chapter highlights an interesting finding: Although CSAR staff designed Seminar to provide informational support, survey responses and focus group discussions indicate that it provides other benefits as well, such as companionship, validation, and emotional support, and especially the opportunity to meet and get to know fellow CRC members. In short, CRC members believe that Seminar is important for their recoveries, but not for the reasons staff believe.

Finally, Chapter 9 describes the very promising efforts by the CSAR to establish collegiate recovery communities in other institutions through the auspices of the US Departments of Education and Health & Human Services. Pilot programs were established at three colleges and universities, and while one of them has ceased operations, the other two are still running, and at least five other campuses have established programs based on the TTU model and the success of the piloting process. This chapter outlines the common challenges faced by pilot programs, including acquiring funding and the difficulties encountered by pilot program staff, as they struggled to balance the dual administrative and student services/counseling roles required to establish and build a collegiate recovery community. Moreover, as this chapter emphasizes that it is important to build program evaluation components into the structure of collegiate recovery programs. Without good data, the funding needed not just to run individual programs, but also to develop programs across campuses nationwide will never materialize.

Conclusions

In the last decade, the number of adolescents entering treatment has grown faster than any other segment of our society (SAMHSA, 2007). This has led to growing numbers of young adults entering college in recovery from substance abuse. Unfortunately, the number of universities and colleges that has made formal attempts to meet the needs of this population can be listed in a short paragraph. Moreover, of these programs only a few have existed for more than a few years and only a few provide services for more than a handful of students. The CSAR at TTU is one of the few established programs in this area. It is now working with other universities and colleges as these schools establish programs to support recovery communities. There is no research that addresses what type of support services work best in which settings. However, existing research is consistent in two ways. First, one of the most reliable predicators of relapse for a posttreatment addict is continued social interaction with drinking and drug-using peers. Second, today's college social environments are organized around the use and misuse of alcohol and drugs (Wechsler & Weuthrich, 2002). To a young adult in recovery, such environments are nothing less than toxic. To create a safe haven for these young men and women, the CSAR has built the largest collegiate recovery community in the country. The experiences of those involved as well as early research findings, some of which are presented in this volume, suggest that the CSAR has been successful in creating a community that protects the recovery of these young adults. This book provides information on the theory behind this effort, the characteristics of the community members, the social networks and daily lives of these members, and the efforts and challenges of replicating such communities in different collegiate contexts.

References

Barber, B., Eccles, J., & Stone, M. (2001). Whatever happened to the Jock, the Brain, and the Princess? Young adult pathways linked to adolescent activity involvement and social identity. *Journal of Adolescent Research*, *16*(5), 429–455.

Beattie, M., & Longabaugh, R. (1999). General and alcohol-specific social support following treatment. *Addictive Behaviors, 24*, 593–606.

Cleveland, H. H., Harris, K. S., Baker, A. K., Herbert, R., & Dean, L. R. (2007). Characteristics of a collegiate recovery community: Maintaining recovery in an abstinence-hostile environment. *Journal of Substance Abuse Treatment, 33*, 13–23.

Dowdall, G. W., & Wechsler, H. (2002). Studying college alcohol use: Widening the lens, sharpening the focus. *Journal of Studies on Alcohol, 14*, 14–22.

Eaton, D. K., Kann, L., Kinchen, S. A., Shanklin, S., Ross, J., Hawkins, J., et al. (2008). *Youth risk behavior surveillance—United States, 2007* (CDC Morbidity and Mortality Weekly Report, *57,* 1–131). Retrieved June 17, 2009, from http://www.cdc.gov/mmwr/preview/mmwrhtml/ss5704a1.htm

Erikson, E. H. (1968). *Identity: Youth and crisis*. New York: Norton.

Gottfredson, M., & Hirschi, T. (1990). *A general theory of crime*. Palo Alto, CA: Stanford.

Harrison, P. A., & Hoffmann, N. G. (1987). *CATOR report: Adolescent residential treatment, intake and follow-up findings*. St. Paul: Ramsey Clinic.

Hingson, R., Heeren, T., Winter, M., & Wechsler, H. (2005). Magnitude of alcohol-related mortality and morbidity among U.S. college students ages 18–24: Changes from 1998–2001. *Annual Review of Public Health, 26*, 259–279.

Humphries, K. (2004). *Circles of recovery: Self-help organizations for addicts*. Cambridge, UK: Cambridge University Press.

Maruna, S. (2001). *Making good: How ex-convicts reform and rebuild their lives*. Washington, DC: American Psychological Association.

National Center on Addiction and Substance Abuse at Columbia University. (2007). *Wasting the best and the brightest: Substance abuse at America's colleges and universities*. Washington, DC: CASA.

Perkins, H. W. (2002). Social norms and the prevention of alcohol misuse in collegiate contexts. *Journal of Studies on Alcohol, 14*, 164–172.

Presley, C. A., Meilman, P. W., & Leichliter, J. S. (2002). College factors that influence drinking. *Journal of Studies on Alcohol, 14*, 82–90.

Rutgers University Health Services. (2001). *Recovery housing: Support sobriety success.* Camden, NJ: Brochure.

Salzer, M. S. (2002). *Best practice guidelines for consumer-delivered services.* Unpublished document, Behavioral health Recovery Management Project, Bloomington, IL.

Substance Abuse Mental Health Services Administration. (2007). *2006 National survey on drug use and health: Detailed tables.* Rockville, MD: Substance Abuse and Mental Health Services Administration, Office of Applied Studies, 2007. Available at http://www.oas.samhsa.gov/NSDUH/2k6NSDUH/tabs/LOTSect2pe.htm#AlcAge .

Substance Abuse and Mental Health Services Administration. (2008). *National survey on drug use and health: 2007 tables.* Rockville, MD: Substance Abuse and Mental Health Services Administration, Office of Applied Studies. Available at http://www.oas.samhsa.gov/NSDUH/2k7NSDUH/tabs/Sect4peTabs1to16.htm#Tab4.6B

Schulenberg, J. E., & Maggs, J. L. (2002). A developmental perspective on alcohol use and heavy drinking during adolescence and the transition to young adulthood. *Journal of Studies on Alcohol, 14*, 54–70.

Vaillant, G. E. (2005). Alcoholics Anonymous: Cult or cure? *Australian and New Zealand Journal of Psychiatry, 39*, 431–436.

Wechsler, H., & Weuthrich, B. (2002). *Dying to drink: Confronting binge drinking on college campuses.* New York: St. Martin's Press.

Zywiak, W., Longabaugh, R., & Wirtz, P. (2002). Decomposing the relationships between pre-treatment social network characteristics and alcohol treatment outcome. *Journal of Studies on Alcohol, 63*, 114–121.

Chapter 2
Collegiate Recovery Communities: What They Are and How They Support Recovery

Kitty S. Harris, Amanda Baker, and H. Harrington Cleveland

Nearly 2 million American men and women are annually treated for substance abuse (SAMHSA, 2002). Unfortunately, as most substance abuse patients will relapse within a year or even within the first few months (Weisner, Matzger, & Kaskutas, 2002; Bond, Kaskutas, & Weisner, 2003), it is clear that treatment alone does not translate into long-term abstinence. What appears to help many but certainly not all of those wishing to remain abstinent is affiliating with mutual help support groups, such as Alcoholics Anonymous (AA) or Narcotics Anonymous (NA) (Emrick, Tonigan, Montgomery, & Little, 1993; Tonigan, Miller, & Connors, 2000; Tonigan, Tocova, & Miller, 1996).

By associating with 12-step groups, those wishing to remain abstinent surround themselves with both the social support of other "recovering" addicts and an organized worldview represented by the 12 steps. By providing the social support of other "recovering" addicts, 12-step groups provide what has been termed "fellowship" (Humphreys, 2004, p. 38). This fellowship of abstinent friends appears to be protective in two ways: first by providing potential abstinence-supportive replacements for old substance using friends (Humphreys & Noke, 1997) and second by insulating against the influences of substance use triggers, such as work and relationship stress (Bond et al., 2003). By providing the 12 steps and examples of men and women with life histories similar to their own who are successfully using these steps to recover from their addictions, AA and NA provide affiliating members with self-support methods and examples for sustaining abstinence from substance use behaviors, improving moral character, and fostering personal growth (Humphreys, 2004, p. 38).

In the last two decades greater and greater numbers of adolescents have been admitted to treatment in the U.S., increasing 65% from 1992 to 2002 compared to only 23% for the general population (SAMHSA). This trend has created a growing population of young adults in recovery from substance abuse, most of whom, because of their age and educational difficulties associated with their earlier

K.S. Harris (✉)
Texas Tech University, Lubbock, TX, USA
e-mail: kitty.s.harris@ttu.edu

H.H. Cleveland et al. (eds.), *Substance Abuse Recovery in College*, Advancing
Responsible Adolescent Development, DOI 10.1007/978-1-4419-1767-6_2,
© Springer Science+Business Media, LLC 2010

substance use, have not completed their higher education. Unfortunately, due to the contrast between their age and developmental level (see Chapter 3 by M. Russell et al., this volume) and the middle-age focus of 12-step groups, the support provided by affiliating with conventional 12-step groups alone may not provide these young adult recovering addicts with the insulation and support they need to maintain abstinence and build strong recoveries while simultaneously growing into developmental mature young adults.

To meet the needs of this growing population of recovering young adults as they pursue their educations, several colleges and universities have developed collegiate recovery communities to help young adults in recovery maintain their abstinence while pursuing their educations. The primary goal of these communities is to provide a safe haven for young adult students who are struggling to maintain their hard-won abstinence while surrounded by the frequent and heavy drinking that defines the social contexts of American college campuses (Schulenberg & Maggs, 2002). It is hard to imagine a situation that could be more hostile to the abstinence of young adults who are trying to maintain their recovery from substance abuse.

This chapter examines the role of recovery communities in a collegiate setting, reviews existing models of recovery-oriented programs in higher education, and provides detailed information about the structural support provided for the Collegiate Recovery Community at Texas Tech University by the Center for Study of Addiction and Recovery. Presenting information on the range of collegiate recovery communities provides a framework to consider subsequent information about the theory, culture, and characteristics that guide and define the two entities that work together at TTU to create a safe haven for recovering students within the context of a large university. These two entities are the Center for Study of Addiction and Recovery (the CSAR), which is staffed by university employees and provides both administrative assistance and financial support for students in recovery, and the Collegiate Recovery Community (CRC) itself, which is made up of nearly 80 young adult students, all with extensive histories of substance abuse or other addictions, most of whom have had long-term inpatient treatment, and all of whom are now in recovery from substance abuse (See Chapter 4 for details on community members' addictive pasts and treatment histories). Included in the community are several members whose primary addiction is related to food, but who adhere to a substance-free 12-step lifestyle.

The Role of Recovery Support Services in a Collegiate Setting

Outside of the college setting, it has been recognized that the recovery success of adolescents and young adults hinges upon treatment and recovery support services that go considerably beyond responding to individuals' alcohol or drug use (Newburn, 1999). To be successful, recovery support services need to integrate addicted individuals into society at both micro- (interpersonal relationships) and macro- (community involvement) levels. A major challenge is getting such integrated services to young adults, who often lack the resources to access such long-term recovery programs. An answer to this challenge is creating integrated recovery support programs within environments where young adults are normally found. College is such an environment. By building these resources in college environments, recovery support has the best opportunity to reach those in need of these services.

The Individual Impact on Recovering Students

Making the college environment into a reasonably safe place to someone in recovery to enter, let alone a place that could nurture their recovery, is no easy task. The primary challenge is the overwhelming lack of peer support for abstinence in these environments. Within an environment that creates serious problems for the average (non-dependent) student, young adults in recovery have a difficult time either finding or developing a social niche that is substance free. Ironically, even normative self-disclosure with non-dependent peers, which would conventionally lead to developing friendships, can create social distance between themselves and these potential friends, leaving them more socially isolated than before. This situation can leave recovering students with two choices: Not disclose and expose themselves to a constant barrage of pressures and opportunities to use substances or disclose and risk experiencing social isolation that could bring about feelings reminiscent of those that led them into adolescent use years ago.

The goal of a collegiate recovery community is to support and value recovery by providing a safe haven from the relapse threats endemic to the college social environment and provide fellowship from others in recovery. Based on a community-reinforcement approach, its goal is to insulate members from positive reinforcement for drinking and using substances while providing positive reinforcement for sobriety. For recovery support programs in a collegiate setting to be successful, community members must see their lives as more rewarding through abstinence than through active use (Miller, Meyers, & Hiller-Sturmhofel, 1999). In order for community members to make this shift, social rewards are necessary. A primary reward that the community can offer is a sense of belonging. Like members of all groups, it is possible for members of recovery communities to achieve a sense of belonging and connectedness to the community regardless of other differences between them. What makes achieving this sense of belonging more likely in a collegiate recovery community is the larger 12-step community's tradition of sharing personal stories of recovery. These stories provide members opportunities to find similarities among themselves and develop a sense of trust and connectedness with all the members of the community.

In addition to social acceptance by and connection to a group, recovery support services in higher education take an active role in providing or otherwise guiding members toward substance-free, yet otherwise developmentally appropriate, recreational activities. This can be challenging during the college years, as many social activities occur in drinking/drug using contexts and many social interactions are facilitated by alcohol (Schulenberg & Maggs, 2002). For abstaining individuals with histories of substance dependency, the alcohol-saturated recreational activities offered by a collegiate environment are extremely threatening. Without the alternative of substance-free activities, the options for safe recreation are limited, if not nonexistent.

It is important that recovery support services in collegiate settings include efforts to enhance academic success. One of the best ways to do this is to implement peer-based tutoring among members of the recovery community. This type of tutoring system is not only effective, but takes advantage of existing peer support networks through which mutual help support groups function. By allowing students who are in need of help seek it from their peers, the students being tutored are able to build trust that challenges can be overcome through supportive relationships. Moreover, it helps them avoid low self-esteem and poor self-confidence associated with academic difficulties that could otherwise threaten the stability of these young adults' recoveries. The students who are tutoring benefit as well. These students are able to witness the positive effect they can have on another's life. By building academic success and confidence and building another connection between recovering students these tutoring relationships help both parties strengthen their recoveries.

In sum, college-based recovery support services value recovery from addictive disorders while fostering a community in which recovering students can grow personally and academically. The ultimate goal of the community is to provide an alternative to the prevalent culture of drinking/drug use on college/university campuses and to ensure that young adults in recovery and those who may choose to enter recovery are afforded the opportunity to achieve a higher education.

Different Models of Collegiate Recovery

While collegiate recovery communities share the goal of constructing a safe haven for young adults in recovery to pursue their educations while building strong recoveries, there are different models that these communities follow to accomplish this goal. These models differ in non-trivial ways. Among the ways in which they differ are their size, housing model, type and role of university staff, and degree to which they apply a conventional AA 12-step recovery model. Besides the program at Texas Tech University, programs supporting these communities exist at Rutgers University, Augsburg College, Washington State University, Brown University, Case-Western Reserve University, Kennesaw State University, Georgia Southern University, Dana College, Loyola College (Baltimore), University of Texas-Austin, University of Texas-San Antonio, Grand Valley State University, and Tulsa Community College. Some of these programs are based strongly on the program at Texas Tech and others follow the model of the program at Rutgers University. A primary difference between these two model programs, and those that use them as models, is whether they follow a supervised residence model, as does Rutgers, or help students find off-campus housing, often with other community members, but do not provide or supervise that housing. The latter policy is followed by the Texas Tech Program.

The Alcohol and Other Drug Assistance Program for Students (ADAPS)

The recovering students program at Rutgers has had a strong influence on the collegiate recovery community movement. This program, the Alcohol and Other Drug Assistance Program for Students (ADAPS), is recognized as the oldest program of this type in the country and offers educational prevention and intervention services. After existing for a few years, this program helped Rutgers become the first university in the country to offer designated housing for recovering students in 1988. The provided housing is designed as a sober-living environment for students who are involved in recovery from chemical dependency or students who grew up in an addicted family (Recovery Housing, 2001). Currently, Rutgers provides housing for between 15 and 20 recovering students in one residence hall. All students are required to attend weekly 12-step meetings and regular counseling sessions with Rutgers staff members who are addictions certified/substance abuse counselors. The Rutgers model has been very influential. Since the introduction of sober housing by Rutgers, other universities have designated sober-living dorms or floors to support students who choose to enter recovery or who abstain for other reasons. Most of these programs are relatively small. For example, Case-Western Reserve provides a two-unit apartment complex for six residents, supervised by a graduate student resident director. Some programs that follow the Rutgers model, such as Grand Valley State University, vary from semester to semester in whether they provide housing.

The StepUP Program at Augsburg College

Another influential program is the StepUP Program run by Augsburg College in Minnesota. Like other programs, it is specifically designed to provide support services for recovering individuals who wish to pursue a college education. Created in 1997, the StepUP Program includes recovery housing, weekly individual meetings with associated staff, a weekly community meeting, and adherence to a contract calling for certain standards of behavior. Students wishing to participate in this collegiate recovery community must have a minimum of 6 months of sobriety and agree to attend 12-step meetings in the local community. One contribution of the StepUP program to other on-campus recovery support programs is its decision to institute a peer government. The StepUP peer government consists of two branches—one responsible for revising and updating the behavior contract, the other for reviewing contract infractions and determining consequences of these infractions. Governing board participants are selected by StepUP staff (StepUP Program, 2008). Since the adoption of this governance system, other collegiate recovery communities, including the Collegiate Recovery Community at Texas Tech University, have adopted some form of peer government system and have adapted the StepUP behavior contract to meet their individual program needs. In 2007, the StepUP Program was awarded grant funding from the State of Minnesota to assist other Minnesota institutions of higher education to implement recovery support programs on their campuses. As a result of this award, College of St. Scholastica, also in Minnesota, is developing its own collegiate recovery community program.

The Center for the Study of Addiction and Recovery (CSAR) at Texas Tech University

The Center for the Study of Addiction and Recovery (CSAR), which is administratively located within the TTU College of Human Sciences, has developed a comprehensive community support and relapse prevention model for students recovering from alcohol and other drug addictions. This model is specifically developed for the collegiate setting and has been used at TTU for over 20 years. The primary focus of the CSAR is to create a comprehensive recovery support and addictions education program for students on the campus of TTU. The program and the community it supports are designed to provide university students with a holistic approach to alcohol and other drug recoveries.

History of the organization. The CSAR was created in 1986 for two main purposes: (1) to provide a unique recovery support and relapse prevention program targeted specifically at high-risk drinkers/drug users and alcohol-/drug-dependent individuals and (2) to provide an educational curriculum at TTU that met the state requirements for licensure as a chemical dependency counselor. Early in 1986, the Substance Abuse Studies interdisciplinary minor curriculum offered the first classes on the TTU campus to students interested in learning more about substance abuse and addiction. These classes, while popular with many students, drew a high concentration of students who had struggled with substance abuse and dependency. Motivated by students in these classes who came forth to explain that they felt isolated on campus, the faculty teaching these classes realized they could make a positive impact on the lives of recovery students by starting a collegiate recovery community and a faculty-run organization to support the community, which was first known as Academic Aftercare for Addicted Students.

Since its beginning in 1986, the CSAR has worked to improve and increase the quality and quantity of the services that it offers to recovering students on the TTU campus. The CSAR has grown in four key areas: (1) an increase in the quality and quantity of services offered to students who wish to desist their drinking/drug using behavior, (2) further development of the Substance Abuse Studies minor curriculum, now titled Addictive Disorders and Recovery Studies (ADRS), to include classes in the general education curriculum for the university, (3) addition of faculty and student-staffed outreach that provides mentoring and positive peer support programs [e.g., Pre-Adolescent Support Services (PASS) and Supportive Adolescent Services (SAS)] to the local school system, and (4) allocation of faculty time and resources to document and evaluate the services offered by the CSAR.

As shown in Fig. 2.1, the CSAR is a multifaceted, campus- and community-based organization. Though it began as a grassroot organization supported by one recovering faculty member, the programs administered by the CSAR are now supported by four affiliated faculty, seven full-time staff members, numerous undergraduate and graduate students, and volunteers.

The Collegiate Recovery Community (CRC). The primary mission of the CSAR is the support of the Collegiate Recovery Community at TTU. While this community has been in existence for 20 years, it has grown substantially along with the CSAR during the last 6 years. Over this time, the number of students who are active members of the CRC has grown from 36, in the spring of 2002, to 75 students in the fall of 2008. This growth has required that the CSAR acquire additional physical space for the student drop-in center, as well as other programs (such as the prevention programs it runs in the local school district). The new facility was moved into in August 2006. This facility provides 9,000 sq. ft recreation area designed for the CRC members. Based on the growth over the last 6 years, CRC membership should climb to well over 100 students by the fall of 2010.

Administrative interaction with the university. Recovery support programs in higher education are located in one of the three administrative areas: (1) student health services (e.g., the ADAPS program), (2) student services or campus life (e.g., the StepUP Program), or (3) an academic college or department (e.g., the CSAR). Unlike some other collegiate recovery communities that are overseen by their university's student health services, the administrative oversight of the CSAR comes from an academic college within the university. Being associated with an academic college has been helpful to the CSAR in providing access to graduate students and building collaborations with academic faculty for assistance with research projects. These research projects provide feedback for the CSAR, as it further develops its programming. Specific findings from these research projects are presented in other chapters of this book.

Primary Components of the CSAR Program

The relationships between the CSAR and both the CRC organization and individual CRC members are structured by six components of the CSAR program. Together these components detail the roles and obligations of individual CRC members, provide structure for the community as a whole, both in terms of its general culture and obligations to its members, and specify the relationship between the CSAR and CRC.

The first of these program components is the requirement that CRC members enroll and attend a 1-h seminar class each semester. The formal title of this course is Community Service Seminar, but it is known simply as Seminar by CRC members.

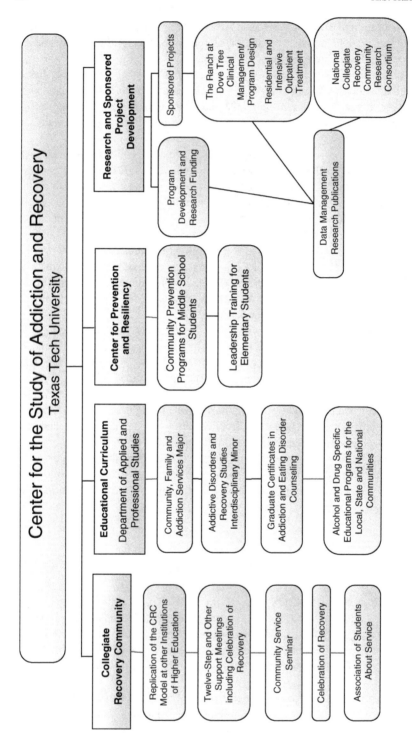

Fig. 2.1 Organizational Structure of Center for the Study of Addiction and Recovery

This component provides one of the most important links between the CSAR itself and the CRC membership. Multiple sections of this seminar are offered every semester, and all members of the CRC are required to register each semester. This class is designed to provide an arena in which members can receive feedback and guidance from peers on recovery and academic issues within a staff-supervised environment. Additionally, it helps foster relationships among CRC members and makes them accountable to a group of their peers within a context supervised by CSAR faculty and staff.

The second program component is the requirement that CRC members participate in mutual help support groups. Although the CSAR does not dictate 12-step principles to the exclusion of other approaches, the CRC is strongly influenced by 12-step culture, at the minimum embracing the fundamental role of mutual help support groups as an integral part of sustained recovery. There are numerous 12-step and other support group meetings held each day of the week on the Texas Tech Campus, these include the following groups: Alcoholics Anonymous (AA), Spanish Speaking (AA), Narcotics Anonymous (NA), Eating Disorders Acnonymous (EDA), Alanon, Sex and Love Addicts Anonymous (SLAA), Codependents of Sex Addicts Anonymous (COSA), and several gender-specific support groups. It is important to emphasize that the CSAR staff ensure the availability of physical space to these meetings, but they are not conducted by the CSAR staff. Rather they are organized by members of the CRC, as well as by members of the university and local community not formally associated with the CSAR or CRC, along the lines of conventional support group meetings.

The third organizational principle is the requirement that CRC governs itself with its own student organization, the Association of Students About Service (ASAS). Working with the CSAR staff, the CRC has developed this student organization specifically for individuals choosing to abstain from substance use who wish to contribute positively to both the university and the local community. It is recognized as a formal student organization by the university's Student Government Association. One of its primary goals is to give back to the community through service projects, such as participating in clothing drives for local half-way houses and homeless shelters, supporting local drug-free youth rallies, and working with university-wide service projects. Additionally, ASAS is responsible for organizing substance-free and recovery-oriented recreational activities. This organization meets weekly to plan events and activities that will help CRC members build a stronger recovery through involvement with the university campus and larger community.

The fourth component is the Celebration of Recovery. Celebration of Recovery is a weekly meeting run by the CRC and organized around the format of a 12-step meeting, though it is not specifically aligned with any specific 12-step fellowship. The format of the meeting is similar to a birthday/speaker meeting and recognizes all types of recovery. The recovery philosophy of the program is open to different addictions, believing that recovery from all types of addiction involves the same processes. Held each Thursday evening, each meeting allows members of the CRC and other supportive members of the Texas Tech and Lubbock communities to come together to celebrate recovery milestones in individuals' lives. By welcoming people of all addictions, as well as supportive members of the non-addictive community, the Celebration of Recovery plays a pivotal role in knitting together the entire CRC, regardless of specific addiction, as well as connecting the recovery community to both the university and local communities in which it is nested. Attendance at this meeting exceeds 100 participants every week.

The fifth component addresses the CSAR's position that academic success is pivotal for college recovery. This commitment to academics is manifested in the fifth organizational component: The Recovering Student Scholarship Program. Texas Tech University, through the CSAR, provides financial assistance to recovering persons who are enrolled as full-time students. In order to be eligible for this assistance, students must meet the following requirements:

- One full year of abstinence from their addiction with active involvement in a 12-step or other recovery support program
- Three letters of recommendation from people who can attest to the quality of their recovery and their academic potential
- Meet all admissions requirements of Texas Tech University

All students accepted into the program are given a $500 probationary scholarship the first semester. Following this probationary semester, scholarships are awarded based on the following G.P.A. guidelines:

4.0	$2,000 per semester
3.5	$1,500 per semester
3.0	$1,000 per semester
2.5	$500 per semester

In addition to the monetary award, students from outside of the state of Texas are granted a waver of out-of-state tuition. Although membership in the CRC is not contingent upon scholarship eligibility or award, most CRC students receive some form of scholarship through the CSAR.

The sixth and final component of the CSAR program is the Addictive Disorders and Recovery Studies minor curriculum. The CSAR has worked with TTU and the Texas Commission on Alcohol and Drug Abuse to develop an interdisciplinary minor in Addictive Disorders and Recovery Studies. This 18-h minor curriculum satisfies the education requirements for licensure in chemical dependency counseling in the state of Texas. The minor curriculum is available to students in all colleges of the University. Many members of the CRC choose to take this minor curriculum. However, most students who enroll in these classes have little or no experience with addiction. This curriculum provides several benefits. It provides the CRC students the opportunities to learn more about addictions, licensing them also as chemical dependency counselors (a career path in which a large portion of CRC members express an interest), and it gives CRC students the opportunity to interact educationally with non-recovering members of the college community. Moreover, by educating the general student body about addictions, the courses in this curriculum combat the negative stigma often attached to the addictive disorders.

The Importance and Types of Peer-Driven Support

The overall goal of the CSAR and CRC is to help the members of the CRC safeguard their recoveries while pursuing their college degrees. To accomplish this overall goal, the CRC has been developed to provide its members with four specific types of peer-driven social support. Outlined by Salzer (2002), these four types of peer support are emotional, instrumental, informational, and companionship or validation support. What each of these are and how the CSAR works to ensure the CRC provides them for its members is detailed below.

Emotional support. The college years are defined by multiple challenges and changes. Both moving to a collegiate environment and the transition to young adulthood can be difficult. Such developmental transitions can alter the match between individuals and their contexts (Schulenberg & Maggs, 2002). For normative students, this can be difficult, as they leave their family and familiar friends for a new environment. For students in recovery, however, going to college can mean leaving one's carefully developed pro-abstinence support network behind and entering into an abstinence hostile college setting. At TTU, this is not the case. Recovering students are welcomed into a collegiate recovery community of over 70 recovering students. This social network is tailored to help them maintain recovery. In this network, new students form healthy, intimate relationships with recovering peers who, like themselves, understand the devastations of addictions and the challenges of maintaining abstinence. To facilitate the development of supportive friendships, the CSAR staff introduce new students to existing members, including matching them with mentoring "buddies." These established members provide further introductions to more members of the community and make sure that new members do not feel isolated at the beginning of their college experience. They also provide informational support, which is described below. Matching up new and established members includes, but is not limited to, matching up housemates. It is intended that the social network surrounding all members of the CRC be populated with recovering, or at least abstaining, individuals and that this network operates not only when the members are at the community's drop-in center, but also when they are outside the center at the university and outside of the university. Couched in this way, the primary job of the CSAR staff is not only to suppor the abstinence of individuals in recovery (although the staff members will intervene if they believe a student is at risk for relapse and guide that person toward the help he or she needs), but to develop and support a recovery community that, in turn, supports the recovery of its members.

Instrumental support. In addition to the value of having abstinent friends, research has shown that participating in addiction recovery support meetings has the positive influence on post-treatment rates of maintaining abstinence from alcohol and drug use (Harrison & Hoffmann, 1987). The CRC hosts on-campus 12-step and other recovery support group meetings for members of the program and individuals in the off-campus community. Currently, there are multiple 12-step meetings each day of the week on the Texas Tech campus. This recovery-specific instrumental support is wedded to peer support programs for academic achievement that is coordinated by the CSAR staff. Specifically, the CSAR implements a peer tutorial program through which staff members identify students who may be at risk for academic difficulties, such as students that failed out of their first attempt at college, or those currently experiencing academic difficulties. Once at-risk students are identified, they are matched with students, very often ones within the CRC, who are successful in the appropriate academic area. Because of the size of the recovery community, staff is very often able to match at-risk students with student tutors who have taken the same classes from the same faculty members.

Informational support. Because the shift to the collegiate atmosphere can be challenging, the CRC provides a mentoring system for all new members. As part of this system, current members serve as "buddies" to new members. In addition to introducing new members to other members of the recovery community, responsibilities of the mentoring buddies include making sure the new member can find academic support resources offered by the university, ensuring that the new member knows about and has transportation to off-campus 12-step meetings, helping them find and making sure they are invited to substance-free social events and recreational activities, and providing them guidance concerning the specific supports and services offered by the CRC and the CSAR.

Companionship support or validation. It is important that people in recovery not feel stigmatized by their status. While the community maintains a respect for the anonymity traditions of conventional 12-step groups, it has also provided members of the community an opportunity to be heard as equal members of the larger collegiate community. Through the formation of the Association of Students About Service (ASAS), the CRC student organization, the recovering population at TTU has gained formal status as a college-level organization, recognized and supported by the Student Government Association of the university. This organizational validation provides an avenue for recovering students to participate in their community as legitimate members without stigma.

Conclusions

In the last decade, the number of adolescents entering treatment is growing faster than any other segment of our society (SAMHSA, 2002). This has led to growing numbers of young adults entering college in recovery from substance abuse. Unfortunately, the number of universities and colleges that have made formal attempts to meet the needs of this population can be listed in a short paragraph. Moreover, of these programs only a few have existed for more than a few years and only a few provide services for more than a handful of students. The CSAR at TTU is one of the few established programs in this area. It is now working with other universities and colleges as these schools establish programs to support recovery communities. There is no research that addresses what type of support services work best in which settings. However, existing research is consistent in two ways. First, one of the most reliable predicators of relapse for a post-treatment addict is continued social interaction with drinking and drug using peers. Second, today's college social environments are organized around the use and misuse of alcohol and drugs (Wechsler & Weuthrich, 2002). To a young adult in recovery, such environments are nothing less than toxic. To create a safe haven for these young men and women, the CSAR has built the largest collegiate recovery community in the country. The experiences of those involved as well as early research findings, some of which are presented in this volume, suggest that the CSAR has been successful in creating a community that protects the recovery of these young adults. This book provides information on the theory behind this effort, the characteristics of the community members, the social networks and daily lives of these members, and the efforts and challenges of replicating such communities in different collegiate contexts.

References

Augsburg, C. (2008). *StepUP Program* [website]. Minneapolis, MN. Available at www.augsburg. edu/stepup/

Bond, J., Kaskutas, L. A., & Weisner, C. (2003). The persistent influence of social networks and alcoholics anonymous on abstinence. *Journal of Studies on Alcohol, 64,* 579–588.

Emrick, C. D., Tonigan, J. S., Montgomery, H., & Little, L. (1993). Alcohol Anonymous: What is currently known? In B. S. McCrady & W. R. Miller (Eds.), *Research on alcoholics anonymous* (pp. 41–76). New Brunswick, NJ: Rutgers Center on Alcohol Studies Publications.

Harrison, P. A., & Hoffmann, N. G. (1987). *CATOR report: Adolescent residential treatment, intake and follow-up findings.* St. Paul: Ramsey Clinic.

Humphreys, K. (2004). *Circles of recovery: Self-help organizations for addictions.* Cambridge, UK: Cambridge University Press.

Humphreys, K., & Noke, J. M. (1997). The influence of posttreatment mutual help group participation on the friendship networks of substance abuse patients. *American Journal of Community Psychology, 25,* 1–17.

Miller, W. R., Meyers, M. S., & Hiller-Sturmhofel, S. (1999). The community-reinforcement approach. *Alcohol Research & Health: The Journal of the National Institute on Alcohol Abuse and Alcoholism, 23,* 116–121.

Newburn, T. (1999). Drug prevention and youth justice issues of philosophy, practice and policy. *British Journal of Criminology, 39,* 609–624.

Rutgers University Health Services. (2001). *Recovery housing: Support sobriety success.* Camden, NJ: Brochure.

Salzer, M. S. (2002). *Best practice guidelines for consumer-delivered services.* Unpublished Document, Behavioral health Recovery Management Project, Bloomington, IL.

SAMHSA. (2002). *Treatment episode data set – highlights.* Retrieved September, 2006, from Web. Available at: http://wwwdasis.samhsa.gov/teds02/index.htm

Schulenberg, J. E., & Maggs, J. L. (2002). A developmental perspective on alcohol use and heavy drinking during adolescence and the transition to young adulthood. *Journal of Studies on Alcohol, 14,* 54–70.

Tonigan, J. S., Miller, W., & Connors, G. J. (2000). Project MATCH client impressions about Alcohol Anonymous: Measurement issues and relationship to treatment outcomes. *Alcohol Treatment Quarterly, 18,* 25–45.

Tonigan, J. S., Tocova, R., & Miller, W. (1996). Meta-analysis of the alcohol anonymous literature: Sample and study characteristics moderate findings. *Journal of Studies on Alcohol, 57,* 65–72.

Wechsler, H., & Weuthrich, B. (2002). *Dying to drink: Confronting binge drinking on college campuses*. New York, NY: St. Martin's Press.

Weisner, C., Matzger, H., & Kaskutas, L. A. (2002). *Abstinence and problem remission in alcohol-dependent individuals in treatment and untreatment samples*. Berkeley, CA: Alcohol Research Group.

Chapter 3
Facilitating Identity Development in Collegiate Recovery: An Eriksonian Perspective

Matthew Russell, H. Harrington Cleveland, and Richard P. Wiebe

As the studies reported throughout this volume make abundantly clear, the college environment is flooded with alcohol and drugs and a student who wishes to abstain must swim against the tide. For no students is it more important to abstain than for those already in recovery from substance abuse and addiction. Although other factors, such as social identity and social support (see Chapter 7 by H.H. Cleveland et al., this volume), are certainly important to the recovering adolescent, a strong sense of personal identity can help a student resist the pressures, both internal and external, to use substances because ultimately only the addict himself or herself can choose to follow a path out of active addiction.

The most compelling and complete model of personal identify formation and the model upon which most recent work on identity formation has been built (White, Montgomery, Wampler, & Fischer, 2003) is that of Erik Erikson (1956, 1980). According to Erikson (1968), college is typically a time of transition, when young adults, having performed the primary tasks of identity development, prepare to take on adult roles. If this stage is not successfully negotiated, identity may be "diffused," among other possibilities (Marcia, 1966). Identity diffusion involves the unwillingness to exercise personal agency and responsibility (Berzonsky, Macek, & Nurmi, 2003). It has been associated with both substance use (Lewis, 2006; White, Wampler, & Winn, 1997) and failures in recovery from substance use (White et al., 2003). Further, adolescent substance use has been associated with the development of a negative self-identity (Burke, 1978) as well as a self-identity rooted in alcohol consumption (Casey & Dollinger, 2007).

Why is addiction linked to difficulties in identity development? It is possible that addiction itself may delay social and emotional development. Adolescents with substance abuse problems may lose their adolescence to years of addictive behaviors and emotional maladjustment that isolate them from prosocial peers and normative social experiences. It is also possible that adolescents who are already struggling

M. Russell (✉)
Texas Tech University, Lubbock TX, USA
e-mail: matthew.russell@ttu.edu

H.H. Cleveland et al. (eds.), *Substance Abuse Recovery in College*, Advancing Responsible Adolescent Development, DOI 10.1007/978-1-4419-1767-6_3,
© Springer Science+Business Media, LLC 2010

with the tasks of identity development may turn to alcohol and drugs for comfort (Lewis, 2006).

In either case, young adults entering recovery are at risk for doing so without having participated in the tasks necessary for identify development. Without having resolved basic issues of identity development, many of these young men and women are faced with the challenge of developing the clear sense of self that will guide them to productive and purposeful adulthoods. Accomplishing this developmental task while simultaneously maintaining recovery in a social context that is hostile to abstinence presents a substantial challenge.

It is against this backdrop of addictions' interference with the tasks that normatively support identity development that both the transition to adulthood for the recovering student and the goals of collegiate recovery programs, and of the Texas Tech University Collegiate Recovery Community (CRC) in particular, can be understood. This chapter considers the psychosocial construct of identity development, as it informs the challenges facing young adult college students in recovery. Prior to detailing the identity challenges faced by college students in recovery and how the recovery program provided by the Center for Study of Addiction and Recovery (CSAR) addresses their identity development needs, the chapter provides information on normative adolescent development and identity crises and how adolescent addictions can interfere with healthy identity development.

Erikson's model frames the following discussion of identity development, as well as the subsequent description of how the CRC seeks to facilitate the construction of a personal identity that facilitates recovery.

Adolescence and Identity Development

In Erikson's psychosocial theory of development, the *identity stage* stands at the midpoint of the eight stages of the life cycle. It represents the central threshold that one must pass through in order to adequately take hold of the responsibilities of adulthood. Because this stage had become so problematic for so many individuals in modernity, Erikson focused on it more than any of the other seven stages in his framework (Cote, 2000). Erikson saw this threshold as a time for healing previous wounds of childhood and for building future strengths that would enable the individual to flourish in adulthood (Erikson, 1968). Healing and building are feasible during this time because of the moratorium on responsibilities that is available to adolescents. Instead of plunging into work and assuming the full weight of family responsibilities, as was the case with premodern societies, the modern adolescent is afforded some "breathing room" from these obligations (Cote, 2000). Erikson saw this time as a "sanctioned intermediary period between childhood and adulthood, during which a lasting pattern of 'inner identity' is scheduled for relative completion" (Erikson, 1980, p. 110).

Both historic and modern cultures provide structured mentoring and various rites of passage to facilitate development of social roles (Gurian, 1998). For example, in modern cultures, healthy developmental moratoria are supported by pathways that take various forms including university training, military service, Teach for America, Peace Corps, travel, internships in vocational training, or just "dropping out" for a while (e.g., England's "gap year") (Cote & Levine, 2002). During this time, adolescents are at liberty to rebuild deficient psychological attributes, explore new possibilities in various domains, and accelerate the growth of previously identified potentials (Cote, 2000).

In Erikson's estimation, the successful completion of the identity stage gave young adults a "sense of inner continuity and social sameness"—an identity (Erikson, 1994, p. 120). During the identity stage, the *subjective/psychological*, the *personal*, and the *social* selves come together. The *subjective/psychological* self corresponds to ego identity. The *personal* self consists of behavioral styles and repertories that distinguish individuals. Finally, the *social* self is made up of roles and statuses that a person acquires within a community or society (Cote, 2000). Completing the developmental task of integrating these selves permits individuals to craft a viable adult identity that answers two basic yet essential questions: "*Who am I?*" and "*Who am I within the world?*" It is through the iterative process of interacting, responding, and coordinating the psychic self (*Who am I?*) with the social self (*Who am I within the world?*) that the young adult constructs an integrated and viable adult identity. When the individual is unable to find intelligible ways of integrating these questions, the identity cannot successfully mature. Poor resolution of this stage leaves the individual laden with unsettled (and unsettling) identity issues and creates a potential for a cascade of difficulties in subsequent life stages (Cote, 2000). Adolescent substance abuse may be one of the factors most likely to impede resolution of the identity stage.

Substance Abuse and Identity Crisis

Initially, Erikson coined the term "identity crisis" to describe the condition of war victims he treated as a psychoanalyst during the Second World War, patients who had "lost a sense of personal sameness and historical continuity" through the exigencies of war (Erikson, 1968).Although Erikson had initially used "identity crisis" to denote a pathological condition, he later began to use it to describe the *normative* transitional process through which adolescents, having already outgrown many of the functions of childhood identity, struggle to establish a suitable new identity. The timing of this process reflects the diffusion of roles characteristic of adolescence (Erikson, 1994). During this time, individuals have cast off many of the identifying roles and behaviors of childhood, but have yet to find suitable roles for adulthood. Within this period, the individual suffers a split in self-images, feelings of loss of their personal and social centers, and emotional and psychological confusion and disorientation. Experiencing some form of identity crisis is viewed as a universal aspect of development and an important part of the transition from adolescence to adulthood (Wires, Barocas, & Hollenbeck, 1994). Successfully working through such a crisis contributes to the form and structure to an emergent adult identity. During this time, not only is the young person free to experiment with different inner and social selves (Erikson, 1994), it is also important to do so. Thus, it is not ideal for these young men and women to insulate themselves from the multitude of experiences that both create and help resolve a normative identity crisis. Unfortunately, adolescents who abuse substances experience exactly this kind of isolation from these challenging, but potentially beneficial experiences.

Not all substance use need impair identity formation. Normative adolescent experimentation with and decisions concerning substance use can be part of normative identity formation. Thus, within the framework of a socially sanctioned adolescent moratorium, normative use does not necessarily contribute to delay or malformation of identity development. However, if adolescent substance use interferes with adolescents' ability to function responsibly in the domains of school, work, and peer and parental relationships, those adolescents are cut off from the experiences that they need to work through a normative identity formation process. It is, therefore, not surprising that adolescent difficulties in these domains foreshadow poor functioning, as individuals move into adult roles (Schulenberg & Maggs, 2002).

Unfortunately, many adolescents cannot adequately negotiate the storm and stress that can typify this time of delay. Such adolescents do not make appropriate use of the institutionalized moratorium provided in their society, and, consequently, fail to create and maintain a well-formed identity (Erikson, 1994). Part of the problem for modern adolescents is that they are left largely on their own to manage the challenges of this period (Cote, 2000). Compared with adolescents in premodern society, they find themselves in a society with weakened family structures and diffused social norms, where they are given a much greater role in making their own decisions. At a time when increased structure is needed to help stabilize behavior and negotiate the multiplicity of possible social roles and behaviors, many adolescents discover that they are allowed to make their own decisions.

This freedom to choose can present major problems when applied to substance use. For adolescents whose substance use is normative and does not become addictive, the decision to "use" can be understood as an attempt to postpone and to avoid the increasing demands of adolescence. Such normative use can be seen as a technique for managing the challenges of this period. For those whose experimentation with alcohol and drugs blossoms into addiction, however, a multitude of problems ensue that carry the potential of negative consequences for decades. Some of these problems directly involve substance use; others are linked more directly to disruptions in identity development during adolescence.

Identification with and being included in a drug subculture are among these disruptions. By forming close relationships with members of a group that approve of deviant behavior, the individuals' drug use is seen not only as normal, but also as necessary for acceptance into the group. This approval provides members temporary relief from ego discomfort related to their otherwise non-normative additive behaviors, thus encouraging continued association. The disadvantages of involvement in this subculture are that the adolescents nurture their addiction and they miss out on experiences that would otherwise lead them to integrate components of their personal and social selves into a more complete identity (Miller, 2002). While normatively developing peers are engaged in the process of examining, deconstructing, and reassembling themselves to meet the needs, challenges, and goals of adolescence, the addicted adolescent frustrates this healthy developmental process by insulating him- or herself within deviant peer groups. The implications of this isolation from healthy identity development are substantial. Unlike individuals whose addictions took hold during adulthood, individuals who began their addictions during adolescence and emerged from active addictive use at the edge of adulthood do not return to a self for which the basic development tasks associated with adolescence have been resolved. Instead, they enter recovery and young adulthood unformed.

Recovery and Identity Construction

The young adults served by the CSAR have chosen to move away from their addictive behaviors and deviant peers and to enter into social structures that begin to support the completion of positive developmental tasks in the context of recovery. Recovery, especially for young adults, has substantial similarities with positive identity development. Like identity development, recovery is a dynamic process in which individuals are able to come to terms with maladaptive behaviors and learn, within the context of healthy social support, to make commitments to positive social roles. Recovery is actively prosocial, and like prosocial identity, recovery is more extensive than simply avoiding antisocial behaviors. In other words, recovery is more than *not* using. It requires that individuals engage in society in productive and balanced ways. From a developmental perspective, the recovery of process provides young adults a prosocial and structured pathway to move through identity confusion and to construct a viable adult identity. The societal expectations and roles that were avoided and neglected during active use are now embraced and integrated.

One of the substantial barriers to young recovering addicts is their tendency toward isolation. This tendency is often expressed when the recovering addict enters college and is faced with a social context where the use and abuse of alcohol are normalized. In this context, isolation may seem like the best route to protect abstinence. Unfortunately, isolation is the very mechanism by which a negative moratorium is protracted and identity confusion heightened. To avoid relapse in the present while also avoiding the isolation that will undercut the development of a fully formed identity, necessary to help protect against relapse in the future, young people in recovery need social support for abstinence in a context that provides opportunities to participate in the developmental tasks that they may have missed during their addicted adolescence.

Young recovering addicts who are in college often seek the support needed to maintain abstinence from conventional 12-steps programs available in the local community. On the positive side, the social interactions with others in recovery allow them to share their personal experience of use and recovery, see that past experiences have worth, and learn to value the person they are attempting to become. However, conventional 12-steps groups are populated by middle and older aged addicts and are organized around the needs of people at a different stage in the life span. While participating in these groups can be helpful, they are neither designed nor specifically intended to help younger addicts deal with the specific challenges of their recoveries or overcome the developmental delay associated with adolescent addictions. What is needed is a community experience that both protects abstinence and engages young adults in (1) acquiring community roles, (2) stabilizing their behavior and character, and (3) developing a firm sense of ego identity tailored to their specific developmental needs (Cote, 2000). The following section details the ways in which the Collegiate Recovery Community (CRC) at Texas Tech's CSAR provides an environment on a college campus that aids and supports these three essential aspects of identity development.

Collegiate Recovery: Supporting Abstinence and Developing Identity

Texas Tech University has established the largest CRC in the nation. With over 25 years of working with students in recovery, the CSAR recognizes that sustained adolescent recovery depends on both supporting individual efforts toward abstinence and structuring a community that provides opportunities for positive development. The CSAR uses specific programming to create a context that supports these tasks. As more fully detailed in Chapter 2 of this volume, the CRC member students make a commitment to actively participate in community life by (1) attending weekly on-campus 12-step meetings; (2) participating in Seminary in Recovery, a weekly process-oriented group; (3) attending Celebration of Recovery, an open 12-step meeting designed to support collegiate recovery and educate the general student body; (4) participating in the Student Advisory Council; and (5) supporting CRC's community service projects. In the process of participating in these aspects of community, members form interpersonal relationships with peers who are likewise committed to abstinence and to the community (see Chapter 7) and are able to investigate and engage in prosocial roles. The result has been a vibrant student-run recovery community that helps participating members integrate aspects of self across domains of behavior.

Community Role Acquisition

The task of achieving a positive community role is a primary focus of the developmental process encouraged by the CSAR. Membership provides young adults in recovery opportunities to acquire social roles in the community, develop character, and stabilize their behaviors. As normative adolescents become more socially engaged with peers across adolescence, the process of taking on positive social roles can occur naturally. In contrast, the escapist and avoidant tendencies that characterize adolescent addiction can socially isolate adolescents from both their own feelings and others. These tendencies hinder their abilities to both interact with and reflect upon the social world. As a result, they are deprived of external and internal experiences that otherwise help integrate aspects of their emotional selves with potential social roles.

For these young adults, an Eriksonian perspective suggests that forming intimate relationships in the context of role exploration is intricately linked to both developmental growth and maintaining long-term recovery. Many who found time in a formal treatment center necessary for recovery have experienced both isolation and stigma when returning to their families and schools. These experiences contribute to making them feel different and alone. The CRC provides these young men and women an opportunity to explore intimate relationships (i.e., trusting friendships) and emotional experiences with same-age peers who have also experienced similar challenges. Social exchanges inside this community affirm individuals' intimate expressions with others. Acquiring prosocial roles within this community is further encouraged by participating in programs designed to instill a sense of unity and commitment to recovery among members. This unity as well as commitment to others' recoveries provides each recovering student a clear role and obligations within the community.

To extend members' prosocial roles beyond the borders of the "recovery community" and into the larger community, the CRC provides service projects both on and off the college campus. These projects allow recovering students to develop a social self that is not defined solely by their being a recovering addict within a recovery community, but as a productive member of a larger society. Participating in these service projects contributes to developing camaraderie with their fellow students as well as essential aspects of generativity and commitment, important components of later developmental stages, according to Erikson (1968).

Recovery Programming to Develop Character and Stabilize Behavior

Recovery comprises a dynamic process that transforms both primary addictive behaviors—dependent chemical use—and secondary behavioral aspects of addiction. In many ways, the secondary or behavioral aspects of addiction, such as habitual lying and dishonest relationships with oneself and others, support addiction and relapse. The process of recovery gives addicted young adults the space and language to face the various "character defects" (in the language of the 12-steps) that make up the secondary aspects of the addiction. These character defects comprise both behaviors and internal states and narratives. Although the misuse of alcohol is stigmatized, its secondary behavioral aspects can often be concealed from both the self and others, making the underlying addiction appear less threatening. As a result, these secondary aspects of addiction can be as difficult to overcome as the primary addiction itself. The recovering addict is encouraged to construct a "recovery identity" that aids in the process of identifying maladaptive behaviors as well as in the task of developing prosocial behaviors and integrating them into the developing self (see Humphreys, 2004). In this way, recovery promotes both character development and behavioral stability.

The CRC promotes these positive pathways though Seminar in Recovery, Celebration of Recovery, and 12-step meetings. The first of these, Seminar in Recovery, provides CRC members the opportunity to learn and manage intimate expression in a nonjudgmental and emotionally safe environment. By enrolling students with a range of "recovery time" in each section, Seminar provides the chance for community members who have less time in recovery to model emotional expression and intimacy to learn from community members who are further along in their developmental growth. These opportunities allow community members to enhance their behavioral stability in a context wherein they are accepted and understood by their peers.

Because seminars are guided by CSAR staff, discussions can be directed toward developmentally important and sometimes emotionally challenging topics. By setting course curriculum and having staff guide seminar sessions, CRC is able to promote members' character development. Weekly topics focus on issues of integrity, emotional, and moral development. Students are encouraged to discuss family dilemmas they face, the consequences of their past behaviors they still deal with, and the challenges of friendships and romantic relationships. These discussions are carried out in a setting of trust, confidentiality, and honest peer and staff feedback.

Like similar college-based recovery communities, the CRC requires members to attend on- or off-campus 12-step meetings or other recovery support groups. These groups typically center on personal struggles and triumphs with recovery and life in general. The process of sharing the affective experience of recovery among support group members creates an environment where triumph over negative behavior is normative and rewarded.

Often the on-campus meetings occur in the CRC building. Following 12-step traditions, these groups, unlike Seminar, are member-run. Self-governance provides important avenues for community members to play an active role in contributing to the community, which in turn supports their own recovery.

Ego Identity Development

As indicated by his expression: "I ain't what I ought to be, I ain't what I'm going to be, but I ain't what I was," Erikson (1959, p. 93) believed that a healthy ego identity is developed by integrating the past, present, and future in a coherent narrative. The capacity to create this narrative through recovery allows young adults to distance themselves from past behaviors and to recast the past as a part of a hopeful future.

Such narratives need to incorporate the domains of achievement, autonomy, and intimacy. The CSAR program provides support for developing each of these identity domains.

Achievement

Becoming a successful and competent member of society is a crucial task in identity development. The college years provide a transition from the freedom of youth to the responsibility of adult work. A college education provides the knowledge and training needed to be successful in the workforce. Membership in the TTU Collegiate Recovery Community helps its members maximize their academic performance. To encourage academic success, the CSAR has worked to develop an environment within the Collegiate Recovery Community that values the academic achievement of individual members. The primary mechanism for encouraging success is through the CSAR scholarship program, described more fully in Chapter 2 of this volume. Administered by CSAR staff, this program sets grade point average requirements that students must meet or exceed to both maintain membership in good standing and receive stipends ranging from $500 to $2,000 per semester.

In addition to the scholarship program, the CSAR and CRC support academic success by coordinating tutoring among members. After entering the community, new members are matched by CSAR staff with academically successful members with similar interests and relevant experiences, normally upper-class members with the same major or minor. As time goes on, CSAR staff monitor the progress of members and ensure that they are getting any extra help they require.

This emphasis on academic achievement reflects a general focus on achievement and competence in societal roles. While there is a positive relationship between adolescent drug use and typical teen-age employment (Godley, Passetti, & White, 2006), the CRC aims to prepare its members to succeed in adult careers that incorporate their developing prosocial identities (see Room, 1998). Positive academic experiences not only indicate the development of useful skills, but can help members become oriented toward professional success. When members graduate, it is important that they are confident that they can succeed in the workforce. The ability to maintain successful and stable employment, while in no way sufficient protection by itself, provides an important bulwark against cycles of stress, isolation, and interpersonal difficulties that can cascade into relapse (Gregoire & Snively, 2001).

Autonomy

Another important aspect of identity development is autonomy. Autonomy is establishing a healthy sense of independence from parents and gaining new status within the family. Normatively, this process advances substantially during the high school years of adolescence. Under ideal conditions, this process is facilitated by honest relationships and truthful communication between the increasingly competent adolescent and the still protective, but increasingly independence-granting, parents. Of course, adolescent addiction and its associated behaviors, such as lying and stealing, participating in high-risk activities and academic failure, corrode and undercut each of the above preconditions—honest relationships, truthful communication, parents' ability to protect their child, and the granting of greater independence—for the development of healthy adolescent autonomy.

The difficult history that addicts and their families have around issues of trust and independence creates challenges for young men and women in recovery who are trying to develop a healthy sense of autonomy. This developmental task is complicated by the transition to college, which can be a struggle for college students and their families in the absence of an addiction. Among addicted youth and their families, this transition can take on heightened intensity and complexity. Parents of addicts can be controlling and intrusive, often failing to demonstrate genuine warmth or concern, at least in the eyes of their addicted offspring (Schweitzer & Lawton, 1989). This parenting style may reduce college students' opportunities to make decisions that will allow them to show their parents and themselves that they are competent and worthy of trust.

The primary strategy used by the CSAR to encourage the development of autonomy is its residential policy. Unlike other college-based recovery programs, the CSAR does not provide on-campus or supervised sober housing. Instead, it is CSAR policy to encourage members to live together as housemates. This residential approach provides CRC members more opportunities to make decisions about their daily lives than they would otherwise.

The CSAR further addresses the autonomy needs of CRC members by running an annual "Family Weekend." This event is organized around multiple informational- and process-oriented sessions. These sessions are designed to educate family members about both addiction in general and family processes that may influence and complicate addiction. Topics covered during these sessions are pertinent to the development of healthy autonomy. Sessions expose families and CRC members to information on the dynamics of enmeshment, codependency, and diffused boundaries as they are related to addiction. These sessions provide CRC members and their families information and support as they learn to negotiate developmentally appropriate boundaries within their families and start to consider the addicted member as an adult child within the family instead of a "problem child."

Intimacy

A recovery program for young adults should also focus on the intimacy aspect of identity. Due to their addictions, these youth may have come to recovery struggling with relationships with their families, friends, and romantic partners, and successful recovery involves among other factors the development of healthy intimate relationships (Vaughn & Long, 1999). The CRC provides a context in which recovering students can build trusting and balanced relationships in which they share their internal thoughts and feelings with others.

In addition to encouraging the development of intimate friendships by supporting the recovery context of the CRC, in Seminar students can discuss family, peer, and romantic relationship topics, such as appropriate levels of disclosure and how to make responsible decisions about sexual intimacy. Outside of Seminar, CRC members interact in various settings, both organized and informal. The organized settings include CRC events, both at the CSAR (which provides a drop-in-center of sorts for students) and off campus, and service projects in the community. Other interactions between CRC members are not organized, but rather emerge from members' natural tendencies to associate with each other on and off campus. These interactions include time spent at the CSAR, which has designated space for CRC members' recreation and socialization (including ping-pong tables), sharing meals (both lunch and dinner are frequently spent with other CRC members), and just hanging out at each others' apartments and houses in the evenings (see Chapter 6 for details on members' daily lives). By providing opportunities for informal bonding and developing trusting friendships in settings outside of 12-step meetings, the combination of these program activities and organic within-community interactions provide these young men and women with the experiences they need to build a strong foundation for intimacy, avoid isolation, and help safeguard their recoveries.

Conclusions

As Erikson (1968) emphasized, the adolescent years are a primary time for identity development. Individuals who are actively addicted to substances during these years forfeit opportunities to engage and learn from social experiences that would have otherwise contributed to their identity development. For young adults attempting to deal with their addictions, the word "recovery" is somewhat of a misnomer, because at the time they enter treatment, they do have a fully formed self to "recover." Rather, they need to simultaneously learn to abstain from drugs and alcohol and to construct a mature identity that does not involve drug use or reflect a drug-using lifestyle (see Walters, 2000). In a college setting, these largely incomplete young men and women must fend off urges to use substances in a context that is largely organized around and exalts substance use. They must do this while somehow engaging in the social relationships and intrapersonal development missed out on during their addictive adolescent years.

The Eriksonian perspective on the formation of individual identities dovetails with social identity theory. Social identity theory posits that the social categories or groups that people feel they belong to influence their attitudes and behavior. This occurs through the adoption of particular defining characteristic of the groups that become part of the self-concept of an individual who identifies with the group (Barber, Eccles, & Stone, 2001). People have multiple concurrent identities that are represented in their minds as separate social identities describing and prescribing the appropriate thinking, behavior, and feelings associated with group membership and nonmembership. Different identities are activated depending on what group is salient in the particular context (Lennon, Gallois, Owen, & McDermott, 2005). When a social identity is activated, self-perception and behavior conform to in-group stereotypes and norms. Social identity and the nature of the social context are thereby bound together.

In joining the CRC, young people also join a community in which recovery and abstinence are the norms. Thus, as they form their new prosocial individual identities within the context of self-identification as members of the CRC, they have a template to follow, as well as social support and encouragement for this difficult task. Ultimately, as Erikson understood, the construction of identity, like recovery, can only be accomplished by the individual, but the support and group identity provided by the CRC can make a positive outcome more likely. Thus, the CRC provides a context that both helps protect abstinence and surrounds the recovering individual with opportunities to engage in social transactions with peers whose common experiences help reduce feelings of isolation. The CSAR supplements this environment with programming that encourages achievement, autonomy, and intimacy. By combining this abstinence supportive environment with programs to help members develop integrated prosocial identities, Texas Tech's Center for the Study of Addiction and Recovery is able to help members build recoveries that will form the basis of an adulthood characterized by responsibility and integrity.

References

Barber, B., Eccles, J., & Stone, M. (2001). Whatever happened to the Jock, the Brain, and the Princess? Young adult pathways linked to adolescent activity involvement and social identity. *Journal of Adolescent Research, 16*(5), 429–455.

Berzonsky, M. D., Macek, P., & Nurmi, J. (2003). Interrelationships among identity process, content, and structure: A cross-cultural investigation. *Journal of Adolescent Research, 18*, 112–130.

Burke, E. L. (1978). Some empirical evidence for Erikson's concept of negative identity in delinquent adolescent drug abusers. *Comprehensive Psychiatry, 19*, 141–152.

Casey, P. F., & Dollinger, S. J. (2007). College students' alcohol-related problems: An autophotographic approach. *Journal of Alcohol and Drug Education, 51*, 8–25.

Cote, J. E. (2000). *Arrested adulthood: The changing nature of maturity and identity.* New York: NYU Press.

Cote, J. E., & Levine, C. G. (2002). *Identity formation, agency, culture: A social psychological synthesis.* New Jersey: Lawrence Erlbaum Associates.

Erikson, E. H. (1956). The problem of ego identity. *Journal of the American Psychoanalytic Association, 4*, 56–121.

Erikson, E. H. (1959). Late adolescence. In D. H. Funkenstein (Ed.), *The student and mental health: An international review* (pp. 66–106). Cambridge, MA: The Riverside Press.

Erikson, E. H. (1968). *Identity: Youth and crisis.* New York: Norton.

Erikson, E. H. (1980). *Identity and the life cycle.* New York: Norton & Company.

Erikson, E. H. (1994). *Identity: Youth and crisis.* New York: Norton & Company.

Godley, S. H., Passetti, L. L., & White, M. K. (2006). Employment and adolescent alcohol and drug treatment and recovery: An exploratory study. *American Journal on Addictions, 15*, 137–143.

Gregoire, T. K., & Snively, C. A. (2001). The relationship of social support and economic self-sufficiency to substance abuse outcomes in a long-term recovery program for women. *Journal of Drug Education, 31*, 221–237.

Gurian, M. (1998). *A fine young man: What parents, mentors, and educators can do to shape adolescent boys into exceptional men.* New York: Penguin Putnam.

Humphreys, K. (2004). *Circles of recovery: Self-help organizations for addictions.* Cambridge, UK: Cambridge University Press.

Lennon, A., Gallois, C., Owen, N., & McDermott, L. (2005). Young women as smokers and nonsmokers: A qualitative social identity approach. *Qualitative Health Research, 15,* 1345–1359.

Lewis, T. F. (2006). Discriminating among levels of college drinking through an Eriksonian theoretical framework. *Journal of Addictions and Offender Counseling, 27*, 28–45.

Marcia, J. E. (1966). Development and validation of ego identity status. *Journal of Personality and Social Psychology, 3*, 551–558.

Miller, P. H. (2002). *Theories of developmental psychology* (4th ed.). New York: Worth.

Room, J. A. (1998). Work and identity in substance abuse recovery. *Journal Of Substance Abuse Treatment, 15*, 65–74.

Schulenberg, J. E., & Maggs, J. L. (2002). A developmental perspective on alcohol use and heavy drinking during adolescence and the transition to young adulthood. *Journal of Studies on Alcohol, 14*, 54–70.

Schweitzer, R. D., & Lawton, P. A. (1989). Drug abusers' perceptions of their parents. *British Journal Of Addiction, 84*, 309–314.

Vaughn, C., & Long, W. (1999). Surrender to win: How adolescent drug and alcohol users change their lives. *Adolescence, 34*, 9–24.

Walters, G. D. (2000). *Beyond behavior: Construction of an overarching psychological theory of lifestyles.* Westport, CT: Praeger.

White, J. M., Montgomery, M. J., Wampler, R. S., & Fischer, J. L. (2003). Recovery from alcohol or drug abuse: The relationship between identity styles and recovery behaviors. *Identity, 3*, 325–345.

White, J. M., Wampler, R. S., & Winn, K. I. (1997). *Influence of contextual factors in identity development.* Poster presented at the annual meeting of the National Council on Family Relations, Arlington, VA.

Wires, J. W., Barocas, R., & Hollenbeck, A. R. (1994). Determinants of adolescent identity development: A cross-sequential study of boarding school boys. *Adolescence, 29*, 361–378.

Chapter 4
Characteristics of Collegiate Recovery Community Members

H. Harrington Cleveland, Amanda Baker, and Lukas R. Dean

An increasing number of adolescents are being admitted to substance abuse treatment in the United States (SAMHSA, 2004). This increase has created a growing population of young adults in recovery, most of whom have not completed college. To help serve this population, Texas Tech University (TTU) was one of the first colleges and universities to develop a collegiate recovery community (CRC). The CRC provides students in recovery with a safe place and an abstinent-friendly social network, but its members continue to face the unique challenge of sustaining their recoveries while attending classes, living away from home, managing interpersonal relationships, and in some cases working to support themselves financially.

To enter the community, the Center for the Study of Addictions and Recovery (CSAR) requires that potential members (a) have 6 months of sobriety, (b) be willing to attend at least two on-campus 12-step meetings or other recovery support group meetings a week, and (c) pursue their education. After being admitted into the CRC, members interact socially mainly with other community members, rather than CSAR staff.

CRC members must work on their recovery program while withstanding a college social environment organized around alcohol use (Wechsler, Davenport, Dowdall, Moeykens, & Castillo, 1994). In this environment, alcohol use is not only prevalent, it is extreme—with roughly 20% of males and 10% of females regularly exceeding twice the binge drinking threshold (White, Kraus, & Swartzwelder, 2006). College can be difficult in and of itself, but young adults attempting to maintain recovery must do so in an extremely abstinence-hostile environment. The CRC directly addresses the special difficulties faced by these students.

Established in 1986, the CRC at TTU is one of the longest actively running collegiate recovery support communities. It has grown rapidly in the last few years to become the largest of these communities, supporting an average of 64 members per semester, according to data collected by the present authors for the fall 2003 through spring 2006 semesters. And it has proven to be an effective program, with only 17

H.H. Cleveland (✉)
The Pennsylvania State University, University Park, PA, USA
e-mail: cleveland@psu.edu

H.H. Cleveland et al. (eds.), *Substance Abuse Recovery in College,* Advancing
Responsible Adolescent Development, DOI 10.1007/978-1-4419-1767-6_4,
© Springer Science+Business Media, LLC 2010

relapses, defined as students who began the semester as part of the community who returned to active use or returned to treatment that semester, during this 6-semester period or 2.8 per semester. The number of relapses divided by the number of members over a period of time can provide an idea of how well the community protects the abstinence of its members. With an average of only 2.8 students relapsing per semester, out of an average of 64 eligible for relapse, the within-semester relapse rate equals 4.4%. Even when considering that members enter the community with at least 6 months of sobriety, this low rate of relapse in such an abstinence-hostile environment is impressive. This success is a primary reason that the CSAR/CRC program has been identified for replication support by Substance Abuse Mental Health Services Administration (SAMHSA, 2007) and the Department of Education (DOE, 2007).

To help place the success of the CRC in context, however, it is important to look more closely at its members, who, after all, do not represent any kind of a cross section of American youth or American college students. The remainder of this chapter reports a study that investigated in a systematic manner the characteristics of the CRC members, describing in some detail the CRC sample, the methods used to collect the data, and the results and conclusions that can be drawn from them. This information can be useful to drug and alcohol counselors, treatment providers, school administrators, and researchers. In the context of the information provided by other chapters in this volume, such as those describing program theory and organizational structures, it is important to consider the characteristics of the community members for whom this community program apparently works.

Method

Respondents

Participants were drawn from the TTU Collegiate Recovery Community (CRC). Data collections occurred over an 11-month period between March 2004 and February 2005. The March 2004 data collection, which included religious involvement (presented here), and social network and recovery status data (presented in Chapters 7 and 5, respectively), took place over two 1-h sessions. Anonymous ID numbers were used to link questionnaires over the two data collections. At this time, the community consisted of nearly 60 active members, 52 of whom completed data collection instruments for this study. Subsequently, data were collected from another 30 participants, as those members joined the community during the fall 2004 and spring 2005 semesters. The resulting dataset contains information from 82 community members. The fall 2004 and spring 2005 data collections were limited to single 1-h sessions. Because of the shorter length of these data collection sessions, some data (e.g., items about religiosity that are presented herein) are limited to 52 respondents. It is also worth noting that several community members' primary addictions are eating disorders. Filter questions were used to skip these members out of several sections of the survey. For these items, the highest number of responses was 73. Prior to data collections, for which IRB approval was obtained, researchers explained to potential participants that participation was voluntary and that all data were anonymous. Food and soft drinks were provided to compensate the participants for their time.

Measures

Questionnaires assessed demographic information, such as age, sex, ethnicity, marital status, living arrangements, family of origin structure, employment status, and academic standing. In addition, alcohol and drug problems, treatment history, recovery history, type and length of time in recovery, drug preference, substance use history, and individual characteristics relevant to the use of social support were assessed. A number of other constructs and measures were also included in the baseline questionnaire to assess substance use dependency, family dynamics, alcohol/drug problems, and 12-step participation. These measures are explained in more detail below.

Problems Due to Alcohol and Drugs. Four items were used to assess family, relationship, and work/school problems due to substance use. These items were based on items that appear in the Brief Drinking Profile (Miller & Marlatt, 2004), and three of the four items appear in the National Longitudinal Study of Adolescent Health (Udry, 2003). These four items were "Have you ever gotten into trouble at school or work because of your alcohol/drug use?" "Did your alcohol and/or drug use ever create problems between you and your [significant other], or other near relative?" "Have you ever neglected your obligations to your family, school, or work for 2 more days in a row because of your alcohol and/or drug use?" and "Did your parents, boyfriend, girlfriend, husband, wife or other near relative ever worry or complain about your alcohol or drug use?" Although these four items were used separately here, an exploratory factor analysis revealed that each loaded onto a single factor, with an alpha of 0.85. Two additional items, which did not load on the same factor, asked respondents to indicate if they have ever been arrested for driving under the influence of alcohol and/or drugs or if they have ever been arrested for other alcohol/drug related behaviors. Each of these six items used a yes/no response pattern.

Treatment History. Six items were used to provide information about type, intensity, and duration of treatment, asking if and for how long respondents lived in halfway houses and whether they were ordered by a court or judge to attend 12-step meetings.

Drugs of Choice. To both describe the community and to allow for separate analyses according to the drug to which members were primarily addicted (i.e., alcohol, nonalcohol drug, or eating disorder), information was collected on members' drugs of first and second choice. Responses provided were (a) alcohol, (b) marijuana, (c) stimulants (uppers), (d) opiates (downers), and (e) club drugs or hallucinogens. Responses to these items were used to categorize respondents according to both their drug of first choice (i.e., alcohol or nonalcohol drug as drug of first choice) and their drugs of first and second choice (e.g., alcohol for drug of first and second choice, alcohol as first and nonalcohol drug as second). Another item asked whether their primary addiction was an eating disorder.

Alcohol Dependency. An Alcohol Dependency Scale was designed to assess respondents' history of alcohol dependency and alcohol use. The 17-item ($\alpha = 0.90$) scale used in this study was derived from the Alcohol Dependency Scale (Horn, Skinner, Wanberg, & Foster, 1984). Responses to these items, such as, "Do you get physically sick (e.g., vomit, stomach cramps) as a result of drinking?" ranged primarily from 0 to 2 (0 being No or Never, 1 being Sometimes, and 2 being Often or "almost every time I drank"). Prior to averaging the items to create the scale, any item with alternate response range (e.g., 0–3 or 0–1) was collapsed or transformed to be equivalent to the range of 0–2 used by most questions to ensure no single item had a disproportionate effect on the overall mean.

Drug Dependency. Twenty items were constructed to assess respondents' history of drug dependency. Based on the Alcohol Dependency Scale, these items were modified to capture drug use dependency by both changing the wording of each to reflect drug use, rather than alcohol use, and by adding several items to capture symptoms more typical of drug dependency. For example, added items assessed whether respondents got paranoid or anxious while using drugs and if they had gone on a drug binge or spree during which they were constantly using drugs for three or more days. Some items from the Alcohol Dependency Scale, such as "getting the DTs, Delirium Tremens," were dropped rather than being modified. Other items that were typical of alcohol, such as "experiencing blackouts," were retained for the survey. A factor analysis, using a Promax (nonorthogonal) rotation, revealed that 15 of these 20 items loaded above 0.4 on the first of three factors. This first factor accounted for 71% of the total variance. The five items loaded below 0.4 on this factor included the more alcohol-typical items, such as experiencing blackouts and an item drafted to capture marijuana dependency ("Have you ever felt so relaxed or mellow due to drug use that it was hard to do anything?"). Unlike some of the items used for the Alcohol Dependency Scale, each of the items retained for the Drug Dependency Scale had a response range of 0–2 and required no transformations prior to averaging, with a response of 2 indicating the event occurred "often or almost every time I used drugs." Cronbach's alpha for this 15-item scale was 0.89.

Substance Use History. Respondents' substance use histories were measured by 24 items designed to assess the specific substances (e.g., alcohol, tobacco, marijuana, hallucinogens, etc.) participants tried, age when they first tried them, and age when they first began to regularly use each substance. Additionally, respondents indicated which substances they have never tried or have never used on a regular basis.

Family Dynamics. Family dynamics was measured with the 12-item scale ($\alpha = 0.93$) from the General Functioning subscale of the McMaster Family Assessment Device (FAD; Epstein, Baldwin, & Bishop, 1983). The FAD assesses family relationship dynamics and functionality with both clinical and nonclinical samples.

Twelve-Step Participation. The 12-Step Participation Questionnaire (Tonigan, Miller, & Conners, 2000) measured the level of 12-step involvement for respondents and separately assessed participants' working of each of the 12-steps.

Religiosity. Six questions were asked about religious practices, beliefs, and affiliation. Questions relating to the frequency of specific religious behaviors were derived from the Religious Practices and Beliefs scale used in CASAA research at the University of New Mexico (see CASAA).

Results

Basic Demographics

The mean age of community members was 23.2 years old ($SD = 6.2$). As indicated by the standard deviation and the lower and upper bounds (18–53), the community includes a wide range of adults, ranging from 18 to 53 years. However, 79% were 25 years old or younger, and only a few ($n = 8$; 9.7%) were 30 years old or more. Most of these older members had been associated with the community for 3 or more years, having joined before its recent growth. Sixty-two percent of the respondents were male and 38% were female. In contrast to the distribution of gender, the data on ethnicity and marital status demonstrate that community members are very similar to each other. First, nearly all (95%) were non-Hispanic whites. This homogeneity likely reflects both the ethnicity of Texas Tech's enrollment, with an undergraduate population that was 80.6% non-Hispanic white in fall 2005, and the ethnicity of those for whom extensive substance abuse treatment is available. Second, 84% reported being single and never married, with only a few being married (7%), engaged (4%), or other (5%). The low number of married community members should not be surprising given the average age and college student status of the community members.

Less than one-third ($n = 25$) of CRC respondents live on campus. The majority of CRC members ($n = 57$) live off campus by themselves (29%), with roommates (24%), or with a relative or partner (15%). Of the 25 CRC members living on campus, 9 (36%) report moderate-to-heavy alcohol/drug use occurring in their housing environment.

Addictive Substance Abuse and Associated Life Problems

Table 4.1 provides an overview of CRC members' difficulties, including legal problems, resulting from drug and alcohol abuse. In addition, the bottom of the table provides a sample of the items that compose the drug use dependency scale. Participants' responses to these items demonstrate the severity of the problems and level of addictive behaviors from which CRC members experienced prior to entering treatment, providing evidence that they were not just casual substance users.

Table 4.1 Problems due to alcohol and drug use ($N = 82$)

	Yes	No
General problems due to drugs and alcohol		
Family ever worry or complain about use?	74 (90.2%)	8 (9.8%)
Did use ever create problems with close relationships?	75 (91.5%)	7 (8.5%)
Neglected family, school or work obligations for 2 or more days?	71 (86.6%)	11 (13.4%)
Trouble at school or work because of use?	67 (81.7%)	15 (18.3%)
Legal problems		
Arrested for DUI?	24 (29.3%)	58 (70.7%)
Arrested because of other use related behaviors?	54 (65.9%)	28 (34.1%)
Dependency items		
Been on a drug spree or binge that lasted more than 3 days	62 (83.8%)	12 (16.2%)
"Felt things" crawling on you as a result of drug use?	54 (73.0%)	20 (27.0%)
Had "shakes" or "tremors" during or after drug use?	62 (83.8%)	12 (16.2%)
Used drugs several times a day to keep a high going?	69 (93.2%)	5 (6.8%)

Members indicate that addictive behaviors impacted their families, places of employment, schools, and personal relationships. For example, 87% neglected their family, school, or work for more than 2 days because of substance use, while 82% experienced trouble at school or work because of substance use. Their addictions also caused legal problems. Almost one-third of community members reported having been arrested for driving under the influence (DUI) and two-thirds reported having been arrested because of other substance use-related behaviors.

Given the extent of their drug dependency, as indicated by the final four items in this table, drawn from the drug dependency scale (reported as a full scale in Table 4.3), these life and legal problems should not be surprising. For example, the overwhelming majority of the community members indicated that they had been on a drug spree or binge that lasted more than 3 days (84%) and had used drugs several times a day to keep a high going (93%).

Therapy and Treatment Experiences

Despite their youth, but consistent with their substance abuse histories, CRC members have had extensive experience with therapy and treatment: Over 80% have been in formal therapy for substance abuse (see Table 4.2). The notion that their path to treatment was not without incident is suggested by the fact that almost one-fourth of the members had been required by a court or a judge to attend 12-step meetings.

Another important indicator of the severity of a member's substance abuse problem is his or her in-patient treatment history. Before joining the TTU recovery community, two-thirds of community members ($n = 55$) had been to "in-patient residential" treatment at a treatment center or a hospital. Of those 55, 60% ($n = 33$) were

Table 4.2 Treatment experiences ($N = 82$)

Variable $N = 82$	Yes	No
Seen a counselor or therapist because of use?	67 (81.7%)	15 (18.3%)
Required by a court or judge to attend 12-step meetings?	19 (23.2%)	63 (76.8%)
Ever attended a 12-step meeting?	81 (98.8%)	1 (1.2%)

Variable	N	Percentage (%)
Ever been in a hospital or "inpatient residential" treatment center?		
No	27	32.9
Yes, <2 weeks	4	4.9
Yes, 2–6 weeks	12	14.6
Yes, 6 weeks–3 months	6	7.3
Yes, >3 months	33	40.3
Ever been in a halfway house?		
No	47	57.3
Yes, <1 month	2	2.4
Yes, 1–3 months	3	3.7
Yes, 3–6 months	15	18.3
Yes, >6 months	15	18.3
Required to attend 12-step meetings by treatment program?		
NA—I have never been in a treatment program	13	15.8
I have been in treatment, but program did NOT require 12-step meetings	3	3.7
I have been in treatment, and program DID require attending 12-step meetings	66	80.5

in such a facility for 3 months or more. For over half of the community (35 of 82), treatment experiences included time living in "halfway houses," with many (30 of the 82) staying in a halfway house for 3–6 months (n = 15) or more (n = 15). The surprisingly long treatment histories of these young adults might indicate that adolescents or young adults might need longer treatment or some type of posttreatment outpatient care in order to increase their likelihood for long-term recovery maintenance.

Although it is not uncommon for substance use problems to co-occur with other mental health difficulties, respondents were not asked to report if they had ever been officially diagnosed according to DSM-4 criteria. This decision was predicated on several issues. First, the overlap between DSM-4 diagnosis and in-patient treatment, which the majority of members reported, provides a proxy for DSM-4 diagnosis. Second, many of the community members would have been in their mid-teens when they received this treatment. Being diagnosed as minors, they may not have been informed about their specific diagnoses nor be able to accurately recall such diagnosis if so informed.

Alcohol and Drug Dependency

Table 4.3 presents pretreatment levels of alcohol and drug dependency, first for all noneating disorder members of the community, then for four groupings of community members defined by their drugs of first and second choice. Of the 82 survey participants, those who were in recovery for eating disorders ($n = 7$), were excluded from these analyses. Furthermore, not all members filled out the two sets of items used to construct these scales. Filter questions, asking if participants had ever used alcohol or nonalcohol drugs, respectively, preceded each set of items. Among the 75 community members whose primary addiction was not an eating disorder, two members had never used alcohol and three had never used nonalcohol drugs, resulting in 73 members with alcohol dependency scores and 72 with drug dependency scores.

Table 4.3 Alcohol and drug dependency scores by drugs of 1st and 2nd choice

			Alcohol dependency scale				Drug dependency scale[a]			
	First choice	Second choice	*n*	*M*	*SD*	*α*	*n*	*M*	*SD*	*α*
Full sample			73	1.00	0.48	0.90	72	1.44	0.43	0.89
	Alcohol	Alcohol	4	1.37	0.24		3	0.57	0.50	
		Drugs	23	1.28	0.37		22	1.38	0.49	
	Drugs	Drugs	30	0.79	0.52		31	1.52	0.31	
		Alcohol	16	0.91	0.39		16	1.52	0.36	
Eating disorder[b]	Drug/alcohol		3	0.79	0.58		2	1.47	0.19	

[a]One alcohol as drug of first choice respondent never used drugs and skipped these items.
[b]Of the seven respondents with eating disorders, three reported not having used drugs or alcohol, one reported alcohol as their drug of first and second choice, one reported nonalcohol drugs as their first and second choice, one reported alcohol as their first and nonalcohol drugs as second choice, and one reported a nonalcohol drug as their drug of first choice and nothing as their second choice.

Overall, the information in Table 4.3 suggests that community members' histories of drug dependency were more extreme than their alcohol dependency histories. This pattern is first evident in lower level of alcohol dependency ($n = 73$, mean $=$ 1.00) than drug dependency ($n = 72$, mean $= 1.44$) reported in the top row. The apparently higher level of drug dependency pattern is also suggested in the distribution of members across the four first and second drug of choice groupings. Specifically, only 27 were in the two groups with alcohol as the drug of first choice, compared to 47 in the groups with nonalcohol drug as the drug of first choice. Moreover, only four individuals indicated alcohol as both their first and second drugs of choice. In contrast, 31 indicated nonalcohol drugs as their first and second drugs of choice. As indicated above, CRC members are recovering not only from severe addictions, but their recovery efforts involve overcoming addictions to multiple substances and sometimes multiple addiction-related behaviors.

The relative prevalence of drug dependency in the CRC versus alcoholism or eating disorders is also evident in the similar levels of drug dependency for the three groupings that indicated nonalcohol drugs as a first or second drug of choice, with mean values ranging from 1.38 to 1.52. These groups included 72 of 76 noneating disorder members. Low levels of drug dependency (mean $= 0.57$) were only reported by the three members with valid drug dependency data whose responses placed them in the alcohol as first and second drug of choice group.

In contrast to the near ubiquity of nonalcohol drug dependency, high levels of alcohol dependency seem limited to the 27 members in the two groups with alcohol as first drug of choice, with alcohol dependency mean values of 1.28 and 1.37, whereas those naming a nonalcohol drug as their first drug of choice ($n = 46$) reported lower levels of alcohol dependency (0.79 and 0.91). While it is not surprising that those reporting alcohol as their drug of first choice reported more alcohol dependency, it is notable that although high levels of drug dependency are observed across three of the four groupings, high levels of alcohol dependency appear to be limited to those who reported it as their first drug of choice.

Although these apparent differences were not hypothesized and to some extent not surprising, they were formalized with ANOVA and post hoc tests. First, a two-group ANOVA confirmed that the alcohol dependency mean was significantly higher among members who indicated alcohol as their first drug of choice ($n = 27$, $M = 1.29$) than for those listing other drugs as their first drug of choice ($n = 46$, $M = 0.84$); $F[1, 71] = 18.71$, $p < 0.001$, $R^2 = 0.21$. A four-group ANOVA was also significant ($F[3, 69] = 6.46$, $p < 0.01$, $R^2 = 0.22$), with post hoc Tukey tests revealing that the alcohol as first drug of choice and nonalcohol drugs as second drug of choice groups had significantly higher ($p < 0.05$) alcohol dependency scores ($M = 1.28$) than the group listing a nonalcohol drug as both their first and second drugs of choice ($M = 0.79$). Other post hoc comparisons for alcohol dependency were not significant.

Not surprisingly, two-group ANOVA revealed that drug dependency levels were significantly higher for those indicating a nonalcohol drug as their drug of first choice ($n = 47$; $M = 1.52$) than for those listing alcohol as their drug of first-choice ($n = 25$; $M = 1.28$; $F[1, 70] = 5.15$, $p < 0.05$, $R^2 = 0.07$). A four-group ANOVA indicated overall differences between the four drug of first and second choice pairings ($F[3, 68] = 5.78$, $p < 0.01$, $R^2 = 0.20$). Notably, this classification accounted for three times the variance of the previous two-group ANOVA. Post hoc Tukey tests demonstrated no difference between the three groupings that reported nonalcohol drugs as one of their first two drugs of choice. However, the groups that reported alcohol as both their drugs of first and second choice were significantly different than each of the other three groups. On one hand, with an n of only 3, these differences must be viewed with caution. On the other hand, because some members of this group skipped the nonalcohol drug items after reporting that they never used nonalcohol drug, it is likely that the "pure" alcoholic members of the community are indeed different than others in the community.

The bottom of Table 4.3 provides the available substance use dependency data for the community members whose primary addiction was an eating disorder. Six of the seven respondents with an eating disorder were female. Although the small sample size undercuts the value of specific statistical tests, the members' responses (and nonresponses) to the dependency items provide useful information. Four of the seven members skipped both the alcohol and drug dependency measures, and one member skipped the drug dependency measures. Levels of alcohol and drug dependency for those who responded to these items (0.79 and 1.47, respectively) appear similar to the responses of the two groups indicating nonalcohol drugs as their first choice.

First and Regular Use

As the information on treatment history made clear, this community is made up of young men and women with substance abuse histories that led most of them into treatment. Table 4.4 provides information on the scope of and age at substance use that led to this condition. As the "Never" column indicates (with only 6.1%, 3.7%, and 7.3% reporting never having tried tobacco, alcohol, or marijuana), experience with licit drugs, as well as marijuana, is near ubiquitous. Only for hallucinogens, downers, and club drugs did a substantial minority (approximately 30% for each of these drug types) reported not using the drugs at all. Reports of regular use were similar, with 9.8 and 6.1% reporting regularly using alcohol and tobacco, respectively. Three-fourths of the members tried marijuana or uppers, and approximately 60% of members regularly used hallucinogens, downers, and/or club drugs. Taken together, these data present an overall picture of polysubstance use, with very few community members trying a drug, but continuing on to regular use of that drug.

The next four columns of Table 4.4 provide data on which grades the community members were in when they first tried or became regular users of specific substances. This grade of use information indicates that most of the CRC members reported first trying and regularly using alcohol and/or tobacco very early in life. For example, over 43% of CRC members had tried alcohol in 6th grade or earlier, and 39% had tried tobacco in 6th grade or earlier. This early experimentation with alcohol and tobacco appeared to translate into later regular use of these substances. Eighty-five percent reported regular alcohol use in 11th grade or earlier, while 78% reported regular tobacco use in 11th grade or earlier.

Table 4.4 also indicates that experimentation with alcohol and tobacco not only translated into regular use of these same substances, but also preceded experimentation with and regular use of other substances. These patterns are consistent with classic "gateway theory." Gateway theory posits that substances such as alcohol, tobacco, and marijuana tend to act as a gateway to experimentation with and use of more severe substances (Kandel, 1975; Golub & Johnson, 1994; Welte & Barnes, 1985; Kane & Yacoubian, 1999; Federal Bureau of Narcotics, 1965). Consistent with the progressive nature of the gateway escalation, the modes for first use of substances are as follows: alcohol and tobacco were first tried in 6th grade or earlier, marijuana in 7th–8th grade and 9th–11th grade, and other drugs between 9th and

Table 4.4 Drug use history ($N = 82$)

Variable		Never	6th grade or earlier	7th–8th grade	9th–11th grade	12th grade or later
Tobacco	First tried	5 (6.1%)	32 (39.0%)	22 (26.8%)	18 (22.0%)	5 (6.1%)
	Regular use	8 (9.8%)	8 (9.8%)	19 (23.2%)	37 (45.0%)	10 (12.2%)
Alcohol	First tried	3 (3.7%)	36 (43.9%)	23 (28.0%)	18 (22.0%)	2 (2.4%)
	Regular use	5 (6.1%)	3 (3.7%)	22 (26.8%)	45 (54.9%)	7 (8.5%)
Marijuana	First tried	6 (7.3%)	10 (12.2%)	30 (36.6%)	31 (37.8%)	5 (6.1%)
	Regular use	16 (19.5%)	3 (3.7%)	21 (25.6%)	34 (41.4%)	8 (9.8%)
Hallucinogen	First tried	24 (29.3%)	2 (2.4%)	4 (4.9%)	42 (51.2%)	10 (12.2%)
	Regular use	37 (45.1%)	2 (2.4%)	1 (1.2%)	31 (37.9%)	11 (13.4%)
Uppers	First tried	12 (14.6%)	4 (4.9%)	14 (17.1%)	31 (37.8%)	21 (25.6%)
	Regular use	19 (23.2%)	3 (3.7%)	6 (7.3%)	30 (36.6%)	24 (29.2%)
Downers	First tried	24 (29.3%)	3 (3.7%)	8 (9.8%)	31 (37.8%)	16 (19.6%)
	Regular use	35 (42.7%)	2 (2.4%)	2 (2.4%)	27 (32.9%)	16 (19.6%)
Club drugs	First tried	26 (31.7%)	2 (2.4%)	6 (7.3%)	35 (42.7%)	13 (15.9%)
	Regular use	33 (40.2%)	1 (1.2%)	4 (4.9%)	30 (36.6%)	14 (17.1%)

11th grade in high school. These results also indicate a very quick progression for members of this recovery community from alcohol/tobacco to marijuana to harder drugs. Of course, since the so-called gateway drugs are less psychoactive and more available than harder drugs, it may simply be that the progression from gateway to other drugs is more of a socially determined pattern than a causal sequence, particularly since most users of gateway substances never become regular users of hard drugs (Cleveland & Wiebe, 2008).

Further consideration of Table 4.4 leads us to wonder about the environmental factors surrounding these adolescents when they first began to use certain substances. It is clear that alcohol and tobacco are first tried at a very young age. This information is not surprising, because it is likely that a large number of these adolescents or their friends were able to acquire these substances from within their own homes. It would be useful to determine if these early adolescents did, in fact, gain access to these substances from their own homes and how long they used these substances before their parents became aware of their use. Perhaps parents of 5th and 6th grade children have little idea that their children are already experimenting with these substances and it is not until later that they make efforts to limit access to these substances.

Lives of CRC Members

Unlike other collegiate recovery communities, wherein students live in professionally supervised recovery dorms, the CSAR staff generally encourages students to find off-campus housing. As a result, nearly 70% of respondents reported living off-campus. However, 31% live in on-campus housing, which is officially "substance free." Over one-third of these on-campus residents reported moderate-to-heavy substance use among the other residents. That community members who are living in officially "substance free" dormitories report exposure to substance use in these dormitories underscores the recovery risks endemic to the college context.

Beyond minimal requirements, members' participation in community events, as well as how much they work their own recovery programs, varies substantially. Similarly, although many community members socialize with each other both at and away from the CSAR, others do not visit the center frequently or spend a lot of time with other community members. All participants reported that they attended on-campus 12-step meetings, mainly Alcoholics Anonymous (90%), while a sizeable majority (78%) attended off-campus meetings as well. The 22% who did not report attending off-campus meetings did not significantly differ from those who did on reports of on-campus participation, such as attending on-campus closed meetings or the weekly community-wide open meeting.

Despite variation in working their 12-step programs, what members seem to have in common is a devotion to succeeding in school. As shown in Table 4.5, the CRC members are productive in school and at work in addition to maintaining their recovery status. Approximately 23% of the members reported a GPA above 3.75, and over

Table 4.5 Employment and academics ($N = 81$)

Variable	N	Percentage (%)
Cumulative GPA		
3.75–4.0	18	22.5
3.25–3.75	24	30.0
2.75–3.25	24	30.0
2.25–2.75	8	10.0
≤2.25	6	7.5
Employment status (during semester)		
Full time (≥40 h/week)	6	7.4
Half time (20 h)	22	27.2
Quarter time (10 h)	12	14.8
Not at all	41	50.6
College		
Arts & Sciences	26	31.7
Business/Eng/Agric/Arch	17	20.7
Education	1	1.2
Human Sciences	34	41.5
Other	4	4.9
Professional goals (plans after completion of degree)		
Work, no further education	14	17.3
Counseling/addictions graduate work	27	33.3
Professional degree (i.e., law, medicine, nursing or research)	40	49.4
Class rank		
Freshman	33	40.2
Sophomore	26	31.7
Junior	14	17.1
Senior	9	11.0
Family financial support		
0–10%	18	22.2
11–35%	5	6.2
36–65%	12	14.8
66–89%	11	13.6
90–100%	35	43.2

half of the members have a GPA of at least 3.25. This academic success is even more impressive when considering that half of the CRC members are also working during the semester, with 35% working 20–40 h per week. These students are enrolled and succeeding in majors all across the campus (i.e., Business, Engineering, Computer Science, Pre-Medicine, Nursing, Pre-Law, Arts, and Human Sciences). Compared with other majors, there is a large population of CRC members enrolled in Human Sciences. This concentration is likely due to many (33%) CRC members envisioning future careers as addiction counselors or other social service professionals. The disproportionately large number of freshmen and sophomores reflects the CRC's rapid growth over the last few years.

Table 4.5 also provides information on family financial support. Less than one-fourth of CRC members reported receiving little or no financial assistance from their families for educational and/or living expenses. Over 43% of members reported that their family pays all or nearly all of their educational and/or living expenses and over 71% of members reported that their family provides at least one-third of their educational and/or living expenses. These levels of support may reflect the notion that it takes a substantial amount of family support for adolescent addicts to become young adults in recovery who are building toward positive life trajectories. It is possible that the young adults in recovery who are more likely to be aware of, introduced to, or guided to recovery support programs like the CRC are those from families that not only have sufficient resources (e.g., insurance and social capital), but also are very supportive.

Table 4.6 provides information suggesting that community members' family contexts are surprisingly average. In terms of family structure, slightly over half of the members reported that their parents are married and still live together, and another 20% reported that their custodial parent is remarried. For the CRC members whose parents have divorced or deceased ($n = 37$), 30% (11 of 37) reported that the divorce or death occurred before they were 5 years old, 51% (19 of 37) were between 6 and 13 years old, and 11% (4 of 37) were between the ages of 14 and 18.

Table 4.6 Family context ($N = 82$)

Family structure	N	Percentage (%)		
Parents' marital status				
Married, parents live together	44	53.7		
One or both deceased	7	8.5		
Separated or divorced, both single	23	28.0		
Unknown, I was adopted	0	0.0		
Other	8	9.8		
Custodial[a] parents' marital status				
NA—parents still together	44	53.7		
Single	13	15.9		
Remarried	16	19.5		
Living with someone, but not remarried	2	2.4		
Other	7	8.5		
If biological parents are divorced or one is deceased, how old were you when the divorce or death occurred?				
NA—biological parents still together	45	54.9		
Birth—5 years	11	13.4		
6–13 years	19	23.1		
14–18 years	4	4.9		
19 or older	3	3.7		
McMaster Family Assessment Device[b]	n	A	M	SD
Original Epstein et al. (1983) nonclinical sample	218	92	1.96	0.53
Original Epstein et al. (1983) clinical sample	98	0.92	2.26	0.53
Collegiate community sample	52	0.93	1.96	1.02

[a]Before coming to college.
[b]Taken from: Epstein et al. (1983).

The bottom of Table 4.6 indicates that CRC members averaged a score of 1.96 ($SD = 1.02$) on the McMaster Family Assessment Device (FAD). This mean level was identical to a nonclinical sample ($M = 1.96$; $SD = 0.53$) identified by Epstein et al. (1983). In contrast, the mean of 1.96 appears to be substantially different than the Epstein et al. clinical sample ($M = 2.26$; $SD = 0.53$). Thus, at least for the environment assessed by the FAD, CRC members' families function more like normal "nonclinical" families than like "clinical" family samples. The combination of normal levels of family functioning and the financial support indicated above (see Table 4.5) may help explain how these young men and women made it into both treatment and this collegiate recovery community. While the overall functioning of CRC members' families appears to be normal, it is important to recognize three issues: (1) normal is extremely relative when examining family systems, (2) some high-achieving families create certain pressures that may lead some adolescents to substance use, and (3) a number of CRC members do come from low-achieving families and have made significant personal efforts toward becoming a transitional character in their family.

Table 4.7 provides information regarding the religious activity, beliefs, and affiliations of members. No members reported being atheistic or agnostic; however, a few members (8%) reported being unsure of what to believe about God. Almost

Table 4.7 Lifetime religious activity ($N = 52$[a])

Scale (0–2 Likert type scale with 0 = Never, 1 = Yes in the past, but not now, 2 = Yes, and I continue to do so now)	N	Percentage (%)	M	SD	α
Lifetime religious activity	52		1.29	0.52	0.63
Attend religious services regularly					
Never	4	7.8			
Yes, in the past, but not now	36	70.6			
Yes, and I continue to do so	11	21.6			
Read holy writings regularly					
Never	13	25.5			
Yes, in the past, but not now	18	35.3			
Yes, and I continue to do so	20	39.2			
Had direct experiences of God					
Never	6	12.2			
Yes, in the past, but not now	6	12.2			
Yes, and I continue to do so	37	75.6			
Whole approach to life is based on religion					
Strongly agree	14	26.9			
Strongly disagree	6	11.5			
Neither disagree or agree	16	30.8			
Somewhat agree	12	23.1			
Strongly agree	4	7.7			

[a]Original data collection consisted of 52 participants. Subsequent data collections added another 30 participants to our sample, however, the religious activity questions were not included in the subsequent questionnaire instruments.

three-fourths of the members reported that they have attended religious services regularly in the past, but do not currently do so. Two-thirds of CRC members reported present affiliation with a religion (i.e., Protestant or Catholic), but only a small percentage of members (21%) actually attended regular religious services. Despite few attending services and two-thirds reporting no current religious affiliation, over 92% of the members described themselves as being spiritual or religious. Nearly 75% reported reading scriptures or other holy writings at the present time (39%) or in the past (35%). The high proportion of CRC members reading scriptures, which may at first seem inconsistent with the low church attendance and low affiliation with religion, may be understood as part of this community's 12-step orientation. Consistent with this 12-step orientation, 87% of members reported having direct experiences of God and 76% reported that they continue to have direct experiences of God. This type of statement or belief seems to reflect the culture and language of 12-step programs and not literal divine manifestations.

Discussion

Research has shown that while it is easy to detox, it is hard to sustain long-term recovery (Weisner, Matzger, & Kaskutas, 2002; Bond, Kaskutas, & Weisner, 2003). It is ironic that there are thousands of substance abuse prevention and treatment programs but only a handful of programs supporting recovery communities. As well as being one of the first program-supported communities, the TTU CRC is the largest recovery community in the country. Their age (Mohr, Averna, Kenny, & Del Boca, 2001) and exposure to the abstinent-hostile college context place members at high risk for relapse. Unfortunately, because the path to a stable future increasingly depends on higher education, if these young men and women are going to build middle-class careers and stable lives they have little choice but to face this challenge. Unless they can negotiate college with their recovery intact, they are unlikely to achieve the middle-class status and economic stability associated with a college degree, let alone maintain long-term abstinence.

The members of CRC are doing well on both fronts, maintaining recovery and progressing toward their college degrees and subsequent careers. Despite the risks that come with the college social environment, the young adult members of this posttreatment community have suffered only an impressively low within-semester relapse rate of 4.4%. These community members have histories of both extensive substance abuse behavior and intensive treatment. Like many addicts, most are not single-drug specialists; rather, most are recovering from addictions to multiple substances. In fact, only a handful are "pure" alcoholics. In many cases, they have been dealing with substance abuse and the problems associated with it for approximately a third of their lives, including all of their adulthoods. Further, they are succeeding academically, again in the face of an abstinence-hostile environment (Wechsler et al., 1994). Over 83% of members have GPAs higher than 2.75. Even more impressively, over half of the members have GPAs of at least 3.25 and almost a quarter average greater than 3.75. Fifty percent reported that they plan to work toward a professional degree (e.g., law, medicine, nursing, or research), while one-third plan to work toward graduate work in counseling or addictions.

The academic success of CRC members contrasts with the academic and social failure of many adolescent substance abusers (not to mention many college students) and raises the question of generalizability: If CRC members do not represent the population from which they are drawn, can we learn anything useful from this study? The short answer is that while the CRC members may be unusual in some ways, especially in that its members are self-selected, presumably highly motivated to maintain recovery and succeed in college, there are not yet enough recovery programs in American colleges to assist all those who would, if they could, select themselves into them. Like college itself, perhaps the CRC is not for everyone but without it, many young people and their families will suffer far more than is necessary. It would be very informative in the future to employ a true experimental design to an evaluation of a CRC-like program. This would be difficult, as the intervention would have to begin before the college years, because CRC is designed for students who have already been in recovery for at least 6 months and preferably a full year.

But are CRC members really substantially different from other young substance users? In at least one way, they appear typical. As the results of this study indicated CRC members, like most substance abusers, progressed from gateway drugs such as tobacco and marijuana to harder drugs and, in many cases, alcohol addiction or dependence (Kandel, 1975). This present study cannot state how this progression occurred—whether, for example, the use of gateway drugs prepared the brain for harder drugs or whether the sequence was simply an epiphenomenon of the availability and social acceptability of tobacco, marijuana, and alcohol—but only that the gateway sequence appeared to hold (Cleveland & Wiebe, 2008). Because of this, there is no reason to assume that the CRC members' drug use resulted from atypical causal factors. However, the members probably differ from other adolescent abusers in other ways.

One way in which they probably differ is in the large number of polysubstance users compared with the paucity of alcohol-only abusers. As noted in the Results section, very few CRC members reported alcohol use as their main or only addiction. The fact that less than 5% of respondents in our sample identified themselves as strictly alcoholics could be a reflection of a larger trend in society that pure alcoholics, except among older populations, are relatively rare. However, that the majority of adolescents who are in substance abuse treatment, then later in recovery (if things go well), are polysubstance users may reflect the phenomenon labeled Berkson's paradox (Berkson, 1946). This paradox suggested that individuals with multiple addictions are more likely to find their ways into communities such as the CRC than individuals with only one addiction, just as patients with multiple diseases are more likely to find their way to a hospital, creating the impression that the connection among various addictions or diseases is stronger than it really is in the general population. There may well be a substantially higher proportion of alcohol-only abusers in the general adolescent population than in the CRC, perhaps because alcohol abuse is more difficult than drug abuse to recognize and acknowledge among both teens and parents because of the social acceptance of alcohol in general.

Along with their histories of higher levels of polysubstance use relative to the population of adolescent substance abusers, the CRC is probably not representative of young adults in recovery. Unfortunately for the thousands of young adults and adolescents who finish primary substance abuse treatment in the United States each year, the CRC is one of only a few college-based recovery communities in the country. For demographic and family reasons, members of this community may differ substantially from many other posttreatment young adults. First, many community members had the family resources for substance abuse counseling and treatment, in many cases long-term inpatient treatment. As noted above, only 25% of them were ordered by a court into treatment, which means that the other 75% entered at their own or their family's behest. Second, these students have selected their college, in part, because they knew of the existence of the recovery community. Perhaps this self-selection suggested that as a group they are more devoted to their recovery than other posttreatment young adults and adolescents.

Finally, CRC members do not appear to be representative of college students in general. As the community is growing rapidly, it is currently made up of more freshmen and sophomores than upper classmen. Further, it contains more males (62%) than females, unlike American colleges in general. It is encouraging, however, that a substantial proportion of females use it as a safe haven from the larger collegiate environment. Their presence in the community may also reflect the growing numbers of females applying the 12-steps or other mutual help group methods to the maintenance of recovery from both substance abuse and eating disorders.

Similarly, the CRC does not reflect the ethnic and racial composition of the United States, its college students, or the college-age population. Like the general population of those in 12-step recovery, the CRC is largely made up of non-Hispanic whites to an even greater extent than the university that houses it (95% vs. 81%), and far greater than the non-Hispanic white component of American youth aged 15–24, estimated to be 61% in 2007 (US Census Bureau, 2009). One of the challenges the CSAR faces is to help develop communities that benefit minority youth.

Perhaps the biggest difference between CRC members and typical college students, aside from their participation in substance abuse recovery, is their higher-than-average academic achievement, with half of all members carrying a B+ grade point average (3.25) or above. This may simply be because they are brighter than average, so bright that, as many of their parents claim, they were bored with high school and turned to drugs and alcohol for stimulation. Thus, their substance abuse may be a direct consequence of their intelligence. A group of substance-abusing adolescents of more average academic abilities may have had different reasons for becoming addicted, but would not find their way into college. However, the achievements of CRC members might actually reflect the educational backgrounds of their families, who have the ability to send their children into the extensive treatment that preceded their current recovery status. The CRC members might also be more motivated than the average student to succeed, because of the barriers they face are far more imposing than those encountered by most other students. A related possibility might be that CRC members are more aware of their strengths and weaknesses than more typical students, since participation in the recovery program, with its 12-step orientation, guarantees that they do more objective self-reflection than is normal for their peers. Each of these factors may have validity and clearly more than one may apply to any particular student in recovery. Whatever the reason or reasons, it is evident that members of this recovery community can succeed academically in college.

That its sample, the CRC members, may be unusual in some respects does not undermine the purpose of this study. Rather than being representative of young adults in recovery, this study provides a profile of the membership of a successful recovery community. In some respects, the members may have been different from other adolescent substance users and adolescents in recovery from the beginning, while in other respects the CRC programming and community may have made them different. But they are not wholly unusual. Like other young adults, community members come from both intact households (53%) and other family structures. Their families exhibit normal levels of functioning and appear to be very supportive of their education and recovery maintenance efforts. What this study demonstrates is that when young adults in recovery are motivated to maintain recovery, have a supportive family and environment, and receive the opportunity to pursue college and recovery simultaneously, they can be surprisingly resilient even in the face of the challenges presented by the abstinence-hostile environment of a university.

Conclusions

The Collegiate Recovery Community at Texas Tech University is the largest collegiate recovery community in the country. As these data show, these young men and women have histories of severe addictions. Despite these addictions, members of this community are managing to maintain abstinence, build strong recoveries, and work toward their educations all the while withstanding abstinence-hostile environment of today's college social context. The progress they are making, in regard to both building their recoveries and pursuing their educations, should help them live productive and drug-free lives for years and years. They are able to maintain their abstinence and look forward to bright future because of the support they receive as part of the community.

References

Berkson, J. (1946). Limitations of the application of fourfold tables to hospital data. *Biometrics Bulletin, 2*, 47–53.
Bond, J., Kaskutas, L. A., & Weisner, C. (2003). The persistent influence of social network and Alcoholics Anonymous on abstinence. *Journal of Studies on Alcohol, 64*, 579–588.
Center on Alcoholism, Substance Abuse, and Addiction (CASAA). (2006). Accessed September 2006, from http://casaa.unm.edu

Cleveland, H. H., & Wiebe, R. P. (2008). Understanding the progression from adolescent marijuana use to young adult serious drug use: Gateway effect or developmental trajectory? *Development and Psychopathology, 20*, 615–632.

DOE.(2007). *Department of Education: Congressionally directed grants 2005 initial earmark amounts*. Accessed June 2007, from http://www.ed.gov/programs/ope-directed/dg-recipients-2005.xls

Epstein, H. B., Baldwin, L. M., & Bishop, D. S. (1983). The McMaster Family Assessment Device. *Journal of Marital and Family Therapy, 9*, 171–180.

Federal Bureau of Narcotics. (1965). *Living death: The truth about drug addiction*. Washington, DC: US Government Printing Office.

Golub, A., & Johnson, B. (1994). The shifting importance of alcohol and marijuana as gateway substances among serious drug abusers. *Journal of Studies on Alcohol, 55*, 607–614.

Horn, J. L., Skinner, H. A., Wanberg, K., & Foster, F. M. (1984). *Alcohol dependency scale*. Toronto: Alcohol and Drug Addiction Research Foundation.

Kandel, D. B. (1975). Stages in adolescent involvement in drug use. *Science, 190*, 912–914.

Kane, R. J., & Yacoubian, G. S., Jr. (1999). Patterns of drug escalation among Philadelphia arrestees: An assessment of the gateway theory. *Journal of Drug Issues, 29*, 107–120.

Miller, W., & Marlatt, G. A. (2004). *Brief drinking inventory*. Retrieved December 2003, from http://casaa.unm/inst/BDP.pdf

Mohr, C., Averna, S., Kenny, D., & Del Boca, F. (2001). "Getting by (or getting high) with a little help from my friends": An examination of adult alcoholics' friendships. *Journal of Studies on Alcohol, 62*, 637–645.

SAMHSA. (2004). *Substance abuse treatment by primary substance of abuse*. Retrieved September 2004, from wwwdisis.samhsa.gov/webt/quicklink/US02.htm

SAMHSA. (2007). *Director's report to the center for substance abuse treatment's national advisory council*. Accessed June 2007, from http://www.nac.samhsa.gov/CSAT/dirreport/dirrpt083104_6.aspx

Tonigan, J. S., Miller, W., & Conners, G. J. (2000). Project MATCH client impressions about Alcohol Anonymous: Measurement issues and relationship to treatment outcomes. *Alcohol Treatment Quarterly, 18*, 25–45.

Udry, J. R. (2003). *The national longitudinal study of adolescent health (Add Health), Waves I & II, 1994–1996; Wave III, 2001–2002* [Machine-readable data file and documentation]. Chapel Hill, NC: Carolina Population Center, University of North Carolina at Chapel Hill.

US Census Bureau. (2009). *Population: Estimates and projections by age, sex, race/ethnicity* (Table 9). The 2009 Statistical Abstract retrieved on June 19, 2009, from http://www.census.gov/compendia/statab/tables/09s0009.pdf

Wechsler, H., Davenport, A., Dowdall, G., Moeykens, B., & Castillo, S. (1994). Health and behavioral consequences of binge drinking in college. A national survey of students at 140 campuses. *Journal of the American Medical Association, 272*, 1672–1677.

Weisner, C., Matzger, H., & Kaskutas, L. A. (2002). *Abstinence and problem remission in alcohol-dependent individuals in treatment and untreatment samples*. Berkeley, CA: Alcohol Research Group.

Welte, J., & Barnes, G. (1985). Alcohol: The gateway to other drug use among secondary-school students. *Journal of Youth and Adolescence, 14*, 487–498.

White, A. M., Kraus, C. L., & Swartzwelder, H. S. (2006). Many college freshmen drink at levels far beyond the binge threshold. *Alcoholism: Clinical & Experimental Research, 30*, 1006–1010.

Chapter 5
Maintaining Abstinence in College: Temptations and Tactics

Richard P. Wiebe, H. Harrington Cleveland, and Lukas R. Dean

As the previous chapter notes, the Collegiate Recovery Community (CRC) at Texas Tech University maintains an impressive relapse rate of only 4.4% per semester, which means that more than 95% of the community members continue their successful recovery each semester. Although one of bedrock beliefs of the Center for Study of Addiction and Recovery is that young men and women who are part of the Collegiate Recovery Community that the center supports should be striving for a "recovery" that goes far beyond day-to-day sobriety, it is important to recognize that in the midst of building a higher level of recovery, members must sometimes draw upon various strategies, ranging from the psychological to the physical to make it through their day, and their hard-won states of sobriety have to be defended against temptations that differ from member to member. The purpose of this chapter is to closely examine the strategies that they are using to maintain their sobriety and the situations that challenge this sobriety. In addition, we consider "where" members' recoveries are in the context of a well-known framework of addictive change, the Prochaska and DiClemente (1982) "stages-of-change" model. Whereas Chapter 4 explained who the members of the CRC are in terms of basic demographics and members' past addictive and treatment histories, this chapters tells the story of what members struggle with, the tools that they use for their struggles, and how they think of their struggles, as something in the past that they have to revisit from time to time or as a daily challenge that defines their present.

One of the theoretical underpinnings of recovery is the notion that it is not a task that once achieved can be taken for granted. Rather, it is an ongoing process. According to this perspective, adhered to most notably by AA and other 12-step programs, an individual is said to be "in recovery," not "cured" or "recovered" (see Humphreys, 2004). Maintaining recovery is a day-to-day challenge, and recovering addicts use specific tactics to counter the urge to relapse, matching tactics to situations. For CRC members, recovery will continue to present challenges after college.

R.P. Wiebe (✉)
Fitchburg State College, Fitchburg, MA, USA
e-mail: rwiebe@fsc.edu

H.H. Cleveland et al. (eds.), *Substance Abuse Recovery in College*, Advancing Responsible Adolescent Development, DOI 10.1007/978-1-4419-1767-6_5,
© Springer Science+Business Media, LLC 2010

Therefore, members must develop the ability to sustain their recoveries while not surrounded by the protective bubble of the CRC. Thus, it is important not only to understand which aspects of their daily lives present the greatest threats to abstinence and recovery, but to examine the defenses they have developed to deal with these threats.

In creating their defenses, CRC members are to a great extent self-directed. In this way, they differ from patients or clients of an orthodox treatment program, in which specific treatment protocols must be followed. Instead of obediently obeying doctors' orders, CRC members craft their recovery using elements derived from four main sources: abstinence-specific social support from peers and others; "self-help" groups such as AA and NA; clinical and other professionals such as CSAR staff; and intrapersonal will and action. In this way, recovery may differ essentially from clinical intervention or treatment, in that an intervention might be said to have succeeded or failed, while recovery never ends. Alternatively, recovery might map easily onto treatment, in that each is a process through which individuals progress in stages. Under this view, CRC members, who have been in recovery before entering college and who exhibit low relapse rates, should be at an advanced stage of change.

One influential stage model of treatment and change is the "stages-of-change" model developed by Prochaska and DiClemente (1982). This model holds that individuals go through four or five (depending on the interpretation) stages when trying to deal with a serious problem such as drug addiction, from precontemplation and contemplation through preparation, action, and maintenance, with preparation sometimes not considered to be a discrete change (see, e.g., Cohen, Glaser, Calhoun, Bradshaw, & Petrocelli, 2005; McConnaughy, Prochaska, & Velicer, 1983). In this view, treatment ideally results in a more-or-less permanent change that requires occasional tune-ups, or maintenance. Of course, this view is antithetical to the 12-step orthodoxy that recovery is an ongoing process that is never complete (see also Maruna, 2001).

Constructs and Measures Used in This Study

The present study looks at each of these three main classes of variables—situations and feelings that provide temptations to drink or use drugs, tactics used to maintain abstinence, and stage of change—in order to provide a profile of the process of recovery as experienced by CRC members. For the study in this chapter, CRC members reported their ability to use different tactics to maintain their recovery and which situations present the greatest challenges to their recoveries. Where possible, data are presented comparing reports of CRC members to those of participants from other studies.

To ascertain temptations and challenges, the Alcohol Abstinence Self-Efficacy Scale (AASE; DiClemente, Carbonari, Montgomery, & Hughes, 1994) was used. Abstinence self-efficacy is the ability of an individual to resist the urge to use substances, and measures of this construct typically ask respondents how tempted they are by particular situations or feelings, or how confident they are that they can resist particular temptations (see, e.g., Sklar, Annis, & Turner, 1999). The AASE takes the former approach, asking the degree of temptation created by factors such as seeing others drinking at a party or having a headache. Research has indicated that the greater the temptation, as measured by the AASE, the less likely is abstinence (Bogenschutz, Tonigan, & Miller, 2006). In contrast, asking about confidence to resist certain temptations, the approach of the Drug-Taking Confidence Questionnaire (DTCQ; Annis & Martin, 1985), does not directly capture the concept of temptation itself, but instead seems factorially complex. High confidence to resist a particular temptation could result from either inner strength (the goal of recovery) or the absence of anything really tempting about the situation or feeling. For example, someone might simply use ibuprofen instead of alcohol or pot in response to a headache; the headache may present no intrinsic temptation to use dangerous substances. Perhaps not surprisingly, the DTCQ has not been shown to predict abstinence (Demmel, Nicolal, & Jenko, 2006).

To inventory the various tactics CRC members used to combat temptation, this study used a modified version of the Alcohol: Processes of Change questionnaire (APOC; Cancer Prevention Research Center, 2003). The APOC measures the extent to which respondents use 13 different types of tactics. To the present authors' knowledge, no validation studies of this instrument have been published as of the writing of this chapter. However, as noted in the Method section below, the APOC, which is fairly straightforward (i.e., face-valid) and describes tactics such as, "I engage in some physical activity when I get the urge to drink," exhibited good interitem reliability within the CRC sample.

The third construct involved in the present research is stage of change, which marks progress from an individual's acknowledgement of a problem that requires change to actually dealing with the problem. A popular stage-of-change instrument is the University of Rhode Island Change Assessment (URICA; McConnaughy et al., 1982). It has been applied to various categories of problems, including smoking, youthful offending, and substance abuse, and in part because of this flexibility, it has become perhaps the most studied measure of stage of change (Sutton, 2001). While it appears to have good psychometric properties, and to reflect valid stages of recovery (Cohen et al., 2005), it has not been shown to have substantial predictive validity regarding the ability of substance users to either remain in treatment or to abstain. Specifically, in a study of an in-patient treatment program for adolescent substance users, only the precontemplation stage of the URICA predicted treatment dropout (Callaghan et al., 2005). And in a study of polysubstance-using heroin-addicted adolescents, similar demographically to CRC members although not college students, the URICA added very little to the ability of demographic and substance-use-history variables to predict negative cocaine urine samples, and nothing at all to their ability to predict either length of treatment before dropout or, perhaps the most relevant outcome in this study, negative heroin samples (Henderson, Saules, & Galen, 2004).

Examining the Stage Model Among Students in Recovery

Along with describing the specific relapse risks encountered by CRC members and the tactics they use to counter them, the data reported in this chapter permitted a comparison between the notion that recovery is a process and the idea that once accomplished, recovery needs only to be maintained. Specifically, CRC members, who seldom relapse, were asked to endorse or reject items related to action, such as, "I am really working hard to change," and to maintenance, such as, "I thought once I had resolved my problem I would be free of it, but sometimes I still find myself struggling with it." The question was whether members considered themselves to be engaged more in the action or the maintenance stage, which would suggest that either the recovery or treatment model, respectively, was more prominent within the CRC.

Method

Respondents

The data presented here were drawn from the same data collection used to inform Chapter 4, CRC data collections that took place in 2004 and 2005. Unlike Chapter 4, which used data from all 82 of the community members who participated in these data collections, the data used for this chapter were limited to the 73 respondents with usable data who reported no eating disorders. The exclusion was made because the most of the variables considered by this chapter—the specific groups of triggers to use substances and the tactics used to remain abstinent—were not very pertinent to those with eating disorders. Demographics were similar to the full sample: Average age was 23.5 years old and 92% of the sample reported their ethnicity as non-Hispanic Caucasian.

Measures

Questionnaires assessed demographic information, such as age, sex, ethnicity, marital status, and living arrangements. In addition, length of recovery, number of years in the CRC, and individual characteristics relevant to recovery were assessed. Data from many of these individual characteristics are presented in Chapter 4. The measures assessing tactics for maintaining recovery, ability to maintain abstinence and overcome temptations to drink, and attitudes toward changing problem behaviors, which provide the major data for this chapter, are explained in more detail below.

Tactics for maintaining recovery (APOC). Sixty-five self-report items were used to determine what tactics and strategies respondents are using to maintain abstinence from alcohol and other drugs. These items were drawn from the Alcohol: Processes of Change (APOC) questionnaire (CPRC, 2003), which was originally designed to reflect alcohol use only, and modified to reflect the facts that most CRC members, as discussed in Chapter 4, used multiple drugs and that very few used alcohol only. Regardless of members' drug of first choice, the 12-step philosophy that guides their recoveries requires abstention from all addictive or mood-altering substances. Where modifying an item would have substantially changed its meaning or where the drinking aspect of an item was specifically relevant, the original language was kept.

Each item describes a situation or thought that might be employed to prevent themselves from using substances. Examples included, "I avoid situations that encourage me to use," "I keep things that remind me of drinking or drug use out of my home or work," and "I use reminders to help me not to use alcohol or drugs." Respondents were asked to indicate how often they might use a particular strategy to help them at the present time on a 5-point scale with 1 being "never," 2 "seldom," 3 "occasionally," 4 "frequently," and 5 "repeatedly."

The 65 items on the modified APOC questionnaire comprise 13 5-item sub-scales, listed in Table 5.1. As Table 5.1 also indicates, the scales showed good interitem reliability within the CRC sample, with Cronbach's Alphas for each of the 13 subscales ranging between 0.61 and 0.80 for all but one subscale, Self-Reevaluation (0.35). The Alpha for the full scale was 0.80. For the full scale, see http://www.uri.edu/research/cprc/Measures/Alcohol06.htm (CPRC, 2003).

Temptations to use substances (AASE). Nineteen items from the Alcohol Abstinence Self-Efficacy Scale (AASE; DiClemente et al., 1994), although ostensibly comprising a measure of self-efficacy, were used to assess the extent to which respondents were tempted to use alcohol in nineteen different situational substance-use trigger situations. Because all members participate in a 12-step organized recovery that requires that they abstain from alcohol even if their primary

Table 5.1 Modified alcohol processes of change (APOC) scores

	n	*M*	SD	Male	Female	Range	Items	*α*
Overall APOC	73	3.29	0.55	3.23	3.43	1.91–4.40	65	0.80
Stimulus control		3.35	0.94	3.27	3.52	1.00–5.00	5	0.72
Contingency management		3.39	0.83	3.34	3.49	1.80–5.00	5	0.61
Counter conditioning		3.70	0.73	3.66	3.78	1.40–5.00	5	0.67
Helping relationships		4.36	0.73	4.36	4.38	1.80–5.00	5	0.85
Social liberation		3.09	0.79	3.09	3.25	1.00–5.00	5	0.71
Environmental relationships		3.62	0.90	3.62	3.72	1.00–5.00	5	0.74
Consciousness raising		2.83	0.82	2.83	3.11	1.00–5.00	5	0.72
Dramatic relief		2.90	0.78	2.90	3.27	1.00–4.80	5	0.65
Self-liberation		3.44	0.84	3.29	3.75	1.00–5.00	5	0.67
Physical interventions		1.42	0.57	1.42	1.43	1.00–3.00	5	0.64
Interpersonal systems/control stimulus		3.51	0.87	3.51	3.52	1.00–5.00	5	0.69
Feedback		3.72	0.87	3.66	3.85	1.00–5.00	5	0.80
Self-reevaluation		3.39	0.64	3.41	3.34	1.60–4.60	5	0.35

addiction is to other drugs, and because the AASE is tailored to alcohol-use temptation, these items were *not* modified for the polydrug histories of the membership. Moreover, CSAR staff indicated that even among members who do not consider themselves to be alcoholics, relapse into drugs other than alcohol was often preceded by alcohol use. Thus, regardless of drug of first or second choice, the use of alcohol was recognized as equivalent to nonabstinence.

Respondents were asked how difficult it would be to resist the temptation to use alcohol under various situations. Examples include "when I am feeling depressed," "when I see others drinking at a bar or party," and "when I am excited or celebrating with others." Responses were given on a 5-point Likert-type scale with 1 being "not at all tempted," 2 being "not very tempted," 3 being "moderately tempted," 4 being "very tempted," and 5 being "extremely tempted."

The original AASE contains 20 items, but one item from the "withdrawals and urges" subscale was removed from the present study because the respondents in the sample were not actively drinking. The 19 remaining items were used to construct four subscales. The first three 5-item subscales assess negative affect, social/positive temptations, and physical/other concerns. The fourth subscale, withdrawals and urges, comprised four items.

Attitudes toward changing problem behaviors (URICA). The University of Rhode Island Change Assessment (URICA) is a 32-item scale designed to assess attitudes toward changing problem behaviors (NIAAA, 2000). In the original scale, eight items assess each of four stages: precontemplation, contemplation, action, and maintenance (NIAAA, 2000). Because study participants, having actively pursued recovery for a substantial length of time, were already past the precontemplation and contemplation stages, only the last two subscales, Action and Maintenance, were used. The "action" stage indicates an increase in behavioral coping as well as other "change process" activities, while "maintenance" reflects behaviors and cognitions that reinforce existing behavioral changes and the internalization of a new lifestyle (DiClemente & Hughes, 1990). Action items include "At times my problem is difficult, but I'm working on it," and "Anyone can talk about changing, I'm actually doing something about it." Maintenance items include "I thought once I had resolved the problem I would be free of it, but sometimes I still find myself struggling with it," and "After all I had done to try and change my problem, every now and again it comes back to haunt me." Responses are given on a 5-point Likert-type scale with 1 being "strongly disagree," 2 being "disagree," 3 being "undecided," 4 being "agree," and 5 being "strongly agree."

Results

Before presenting details on the tactics CRC members employ, the situations that threaten their recoveries, and where they stand in relation to other samples regarding their recovery maintenance processes, it is important to reemphasize the success of the program in which the CRC members participate. As demonstrated by the low within-semester relapse rate of 4.4% (see Chapter 4) the relapse prevention program provided by the CSAR via the CRC appears to be highly protective of young people's abstinence. It is with this success and the collegiate context in mind in which the CRC members are nested that the following information is presented.

Tactics for Maintaining Recovery (APOC)

Information on the APOC subscales is presented in Table 5.1. All items and resulting scales had a range of 1 (never using a particular tactic to avoid temptation) to 5 (repeatedly). Of the 13 subscales, the mean score for the Helping Relationships subscale was the highest. The extremely high mean score of 4.36 (SD = 0.73) indicates that CRC members reported "frequently" or "repeatedly" having someone who provides social support to their recovery maintenance. That the mean of this subscale is so high reflects the success of the CRC in providing its members social support to aid in their recovery maintenance. The high mean on this subscale may also reflect the 12-step philosophy of the CSAR, as it works to build a recovery community that simultaneously buffers members from aspects of collegiate culture that present challenges to its members while at the same time still allows the conventional social support systems that are at the core of the 12-step mutual help system to function.

At the other end of the distribution were respondents' answers for tactics involving Physical Interventions: Their mean of 1.42 (SD = 0.57) subscale was the lowest of the 13 APOC subscales. The mean of 1.42 on this subscale indicated that CRC members reported "never" or "seldom" having to take some type of drug or medication to help them maintain recovery. Similar to the high mean of helping relationships, the low use of medication to control addictions likely reflects the 12-step culture that generally opposes relying on medications to overcome substance use problems, as this would constitute substituting one form of dependence for another.

Three of the APOC subscales have means that indicate they are "occasionally" used as tactics to maintain abstinence: Consciousness Raising ($M = 2.83$), Dramatic Relief ($M = 2.90$), and Social Liberation ($M = 3.09$). These scores suggest that CRC members "occasionally" look for, see, and contribute to public information regarding the potential dangers of substance use through both the media and their own social interactions.

The other eight subscales had means ranging between 3.35 and 3.72, between "occasionally" (3) and "frequently" (4). That most subscales have means over 3 suggests that CRC members are utilizing a variety of tactics to aid in maintaining abstinence. The means for Feedback ($M = 3.72$), Counter Conditioning ($M = 3.70$), Environmental Relationships ($M = 3.62$), and Interpersonal Systems/Control Stimulus ($M = 3.51$) approached "frequent" utilization. Tactics represented by Self-Liberation ($M = 3.44$), Self-Reevaluation ($M = 3.39$), Contingency Management ($M = 3.39$), and Stimulus Control ($M = 3.35$) were utilized slightly more than "occasionally," but not "frequently," based on the mean responses of CRC members.

Biological sex. A quick look at the mean scores by biological sex is revealing. Before considering the conventionally calculated statistical significance of any differences, it is worth noting that females scored higher than males on 12 of the 13 subscales. If the possibility of females scoring higher than males were random (i.e., each had a 50% chance for each subscale), then the probability that females would score higher on 12 of the 13 subscales would be 0.001587 (13/8192). Formalizing this with a different approach, the significance test suggested by Bruning and Kintz (1987) provides a z-score of 5.724, $p < 0.05$.

It is unclear why the female respondents scored higher on these subscales. Perhaps gender norms allow females to be more open to applying recovery tactics than males. Or perhaps females in general are more cognizant of and effortful in their recovery maintenance efforts. More research is warranted to determine if females consistently score higher on the APOC scale and its subscales, or if the females at the CRC are unique in this way. Only for Self-Reevaluation were male ($M = 3.41$) scores higher than female ($M = 3.34$) scores. Because Self-Reevaluation is strongly tied to feelings and reflexive thoughts about self, it is a little surprising that male respondents scored higher than female respondents on this subscale. However, it may be that self-reevaluation as a process reflects the greater egotism of the male (see, e.g., Baumeister, Smart, & Boden, 1996). Of course, all this post hoc reasoning may be irrelevant, because the finding may have resulted mainly from measurement error: Self-Reevaluation showed by far the weakest reliability of any subscale ($\alpha = 0.35$).

Not surprisingly, with such a small sample size, most of the differences between sex were not statistically significant. The exceptions included Consciousness Raising ($F[1, 72] = 4.30, p \leq 0.05$; females $= 3.11$, males $= 2.69$), Dramatic Relief ($F[1, 72] = 8.65, p \leq 0.01$; females $= 3.27$, males $= 2.72$), and Self-Liberation ($F[1, 72] = 5.05, p \leq 0.05$; females $= 3.75$, males $= 3.29$). The differences for Consciousness Raising (sample item: "I read newspaper stories that may help me quit drinking") and Dramatic Relief (sample item: "Stories about alcohol and its effects upset me") suggest that women in the CRC tend to seek, and respond emotionally to, information regarding problems associated with substance use from individuals, media, and meetings.

The differences for the Self-Liberation (sample item: "I use willpower to keep from drinking") subscale indicated that women rely more frequently than men on their own willpower or personal effort and commitment to maintain recovery. This higher reliance on oneself may not be a positive characteristic: If they were relying on self rather than others, their recoveries might be at risk. However, females in the CRC reported higher scores, albeit not significantly so, on the Helping Relationships subscale as well. This suggests that at least among the women in the CRC, reliance on the self does not preclude reliance on others.

Length of recovery. Using ANOVA, statistically significant differences were found for 3 of the 13 subscales, Stimulus Control ($F[3, 66] = 4.18, p < 0.01$), Interpersonal Systems/Control Systems ($F[3, 66] = 3.92, p < 0.05$), and Counterconditioning ($F[3, 66] = 3.20, p < 0.05$), according to respondents' length of drug recovery. Each of these represents a focused individual action aimed at preventing relapse. The Stimulus Control (sample item: "I keep things around my home or work that remind me not to drink") and Interpersonal Systems/Control Systems (sample item: "I change personal relationships which contribute to my drinking") subscales address how respondents avoid situations or individuals that encourage them to use substances. The Counterconditioning subscale indicates how often the respondent engages in alternate physical or mental activities when feeling the urge to use substances.

Post hoc Tukey tests reveal that respondents ($n = 24$) who reported having been in recovery for between 7 and 24 months have significantly higher scores on the stimulus control subscale ($M = 3.76$) than respondents who have been in drug abuse recovery for over five years ($M = 2.67$; $p < 0.05$). Post hoc Tukey tests also reveal that respondents who reported having been in recovery for between 7 and 24 months reported significantly higher scores on the interpersonal systems/control stimulus subscale ($M = 3.92$) than respondents who have been in drug abuse recovery for over five years ($M = 2.98$; $p < 0.01$). These mean scores indicate that on average, respondents who have been in recovery for between 7 and 24 months "frequently" avoid people or places that encourage substance use whereas respondents who have been in recovery for over 5 years only "occasionally" do the same. Tukey post hoc tests also revealed that respondents who have been in recovery for between 7 and 24 months reported significantly higher scores on the counterconditioning subscale ($M = 3.93$) than respondents who have been in drug abuse recovery for over five years ($M = 3.24$; $p < 0.05$).

These findings suggest that respondents who have been in recovery longer than 5 years either start to become less vigilant in some recovery maintenance tactics, or have already arranged their social and environmental contexts and gained control of their urges in such a way that requires much less present effort in order to maintain recovery. While using fewer tactics might put them at risk, their recoveries may be strong enough that they don't have to avoid situations and people that and who could have threatened their recoveries only a few years earlier. Perhaps their cravings and urges may have grown more mild, or at least less salient, over time so they no longer have to use the direct tactics assessed by the Counterconditioning subscale. There is another possibility that after so many years of recovery, they have organized their lives and social networks in such ways that they no longer have to actively avoid people and contexts that would put them at risk for relapse, because their lives no longer overlap with such people and contexts.

In contrast, the data suggest that CRC members whose recovery is relatively new try hard to distance themselves from situations and people that they feel may threaten their recovery. Similarly, they also make changes aimed at avoiding thoughts of using. It may be the case that relatively fresh from treatment, they realize the need to actively work to protect their recovery and that their reported scores have a mean of nearly 4 on a scale of 1–5 indicates devotion to recovery maintenance.

Similar analyses were performed to consider whether the participant differed by time in the community. Unlike results for time in recovery, participants' modified APOC scores did not differ by time in the community.

Extent of Temptations to Drink (AASE)

Table 5.2 presents the means for the four Alcohol Abstinence Self-Efficacy subscales and the items that contribute to each for the CRC sample. It also provides

Table 5.2 Alcohol Abstinence Self-Efficacy (AASE) scores

	CRC sample ($n = 73$)		DiClemente et al. sample ($n = 266$)		Cohen "D" score
	M	SD	M	SD	D
Negative affect	2.2	1.1	2.6[a]	1.3[a]	−0.33
When I am feeling angry inside	2.2	1.2	2.7	1.2	−0.42
When I sense everything is going wrong for me	2.4	1.3	2.4	1.3	0.00
When I am feeling depressed	2.3	1.3	2.5	1.3	−0.15
When I feel like blowing up because of frustration	2.3	1.2	2.6	1.3	−0.24
When I am very worried	1.9	1.0	2.6	1.2	−0.64
Social/positive	2.0	0.9	2.8[a]	1.3[a]	−0.73
When I see others drinking at a bar or at a party	2.1	1.1	2.7	1.3	−0.50
When I am excited or celebrating with others	1.9	1.1	2.7	1.3	−0.67
When I am on vacation and want to relax	2.0	1.1	2.7	1.3	−0.58
When people I used to drink with encourage me to drink	1.8	1.2	2.9	1.4	−0.85
When I am being offered a drink in a social situation	1.9	1.0	2.8	1.3	−0.78
Physical and other concerns	1.7	0.9	3.4[a]	1.4[a]	−1.48
When I have a headache	1.5	0.9	3.6	1.5	−1.75
When I am physically tired	1.7	1.1	3.4	1.3	−1.42
When I am concerned about someone	1.5	1.0	3.3	1.3	−1.57
When I am expecting some physical pain or injury	1.9	1.3	3.3	1.4	−1.04
When I dream about taking a drink	2.1	1.2	3.6	1.5	−1.11
Withdrawal, cravings, and urges[b]	2.0	1.0	2.9[a]	1.4[a]	−0.75
When I have the urge to try just one drink to see what happens	2.0	1.2	2.9	1.4	−0.47
When I am feeling a physical need or craving for alcohol	2.1	1.3	2.7	1.4	−0.44
When I want to test my willpower over drinking	1.6	1.1	3.1	1.4	−1.20
When I experience an urge or impulse to take a drink that catches me unprepared	2.3	1.3	2.8	1.3	−0.38

[a] Note: Overall subscale *M* and SD inferred from statistics reported in DiClemente et al. (1994) Table 5.1.
[b] Note: DiClemente et al. (1994) withdrawals subscale contains 5 items. CRC subscale computed with 4 items.

comparable data from previously published clinical comparison sample (DiClemente et al., 1994), which will be discussed subsequently. Of the four AASE subscales, the mean for Negative Affect was the highest. CRC members reported feeling more tempted to drink alcohol when experiencing negative affect ($M = 2.24$, SD $= 1.09$, á $= 0.94$) than physical pain or other concerns. However, the means for the other self-efficacy subscales were not substantially different: The Social/Positive and Withdrawals, Cravings, and Urges subscales both had means of 2.0. The lowest subscale was Physical Pain or Other Concerns with a mean of 1.72. The relatively low mean scores on these subscales (2.24 or below on a scale of 1–5) indicates that the sample generally reports low levels of temptation. That the lowest scores were for physical pain may possibly reflect the young ages of most CRC members. It may be that they do not associate risk of use with physical difficulties. But given their age, it may also be that they have not had a lot of experience with physical difficulties.

That the sample scored highest on negative affect may also reflect the youth of most members. These men and women differ from conventional alcoholics and drug addicts in both their current age and the age when they developed their addictions. They may have learned to rely on drugs and alcohol as a means of coping with daily stressors before developing other, more positive means of dealing with challenges in relationships, education, and work. Because such stressors are an unavoidable part of adult life, unlike social celebrations or bars which can be avoided, it seems clear that these young men and women will have to develop other ways of coping with negative affect.

Biological sex. Table 5.3 presents the means for the AASE subscales by biological sex. While no significant differences were found, a clear pattern exists. Males reported slightly higher mean scores on all four subscales. These differences were small, but perhaps it is notable that CRC males may be reporting more temptation than females, considering that females reported greater use of 12 of the 13 types of recovery tactics.

Table 5.3 Alcohol Abstinence Self-Efficacy (AASE) scores by biological sex

AASE	Male	Female
Negative affect	2.27 (1.07)	2.18 (1.13)
Social/positive	2.03 (0.96)	1.81 (0.91)
Physical/other concerns	1.78 (0.91)	1.61 (0.96)
Withdrawals and cravings	2.06 (0.94)	1.99 (1.12)
	$n = 49$	$n = 24$

Length of drug abuse or drug dependency recovery. Time matters. From the left of Table 5.4, which presents the means for the AASE subscales by respondents' length of recovery, to the right, a clear trend exists. On the left are the scores for the few members of the CRC who have less than 6 months of recovery. These scores appear higher than all other groups. As length of recovery increases, temptations associated with negative affect, social and other positive stimuli, and withdrawals and cravings decrease. ANOVAs revealed significant differences for each subscale

Table 5.4 Abstinence Abuse Self-Efficacy (AASE) scores by length of recovery

AASE	0–6 months	7–24 months	2–5 years	5+ years
Negative affect	3.56 (1.26)	2.33 (0.99)	2.05 (0.94)	2.15 (1.37)
Social/positive	3.64 (1.15)	2.00 (0.72)	1.73 (0.67)	1.85 (1.26)
Physical/other concerns	3.12 (1.34)	1.72 (0.70)	1.47 (0.58)	1.93 (1.40)
Withdrawal, cravings, and urges	3.65 (1.14)	2.02 (0.76)	1.92 (0.82)	1.80 (1.24)
	$n = 5$	$n = 24$	$n = 27$	$n = 11$

(Negative Affect, $F[3, 66] = 2.95$, $p < 0.05$, $R^2 = 0.06$; Social/Positive, $F[3, 66] = 7.32$, $p < 0.001$, $R^2 = 0.12$; Physical/Other Concerns, $F[3, 66] = 5.30$, $p < 0.01$, $R^2 = 0.04$; and Withdrawals/Cravings, $F[3, 65] = 5.67$, $p < 0.01$, $R^2 = 0.11$). More specifically, Tukey post hoc tests reveal that respondents who have been in drug abuse and/or drug dependency recovery for less than 6 months reported significantly higher temptation to drink in all four AASE subscales when compared with respondents who have been in drug abuse recovery for between 2 and 5 years (Negative Affect, $p < 0.05$, Social/Positive, $p < 0.001$, Physical/Other Concerns, $p < 0.01$, Withdrawals/ Cravings, $p < 0.01$). The mean scores for those who have been in drug abuse recovery for less than six months were above 3.12 (ranging from 3.12 to 3.65) for all four subscales, and the mean difference scores between these members compared with respondents who had been in recovery for between 2 and 5 years were over 1.5 for all four subscales. When compared with respondents who have been in drug abuse recovery for between 7 and 24 months, respondents who have been in drug abuse recovery for less than 6 months reported significantly higher temptation to drink for three of the four AASE subscales (social/positive, $p < 0.01$; physical, $p < 0.05$; cravings, $p < 0.01$). For both the social/positive subscale and the cravings/withdrawals subscale, respondents who had been in drug abuse recovery for less than 6 months reported significantly higher temptation to drink than all three other subgroups who reported longer lengths of drug abuse recovery.

These results demonstrate something that the addictions professionals and researchers have known for some time: People with shorter recoveries have a substantially greater risk for relapse. For this reason the formal CSAR policy is that members must have at least 6 months of recovery before joining the community and a year of recovery before receiving a scholarship. This policy is not strictly enforced, as the CSAR has admitted people with shorter recoveries into the CRC. Each time this decision must be made carefully. The CSAR leadership feels that while exceptions can be made, the general policy is important as applying it in most cases has helped create a community that on average shows relatively low levels of temptations across these different domains.

Similar analyses were performed to consider whether the participants differed by time in the community. Unlike results for time in recovery, participants' AASE scores did not differ by time in the community.

Comparison between CRC members and a clinical sample. In addition to the scores from the CRC sample, Table 5.2 provides comparison data from sample of 266 adults who applied for treatment at the Outpatient Alcoholism Treatment Program at the Texas Research Institute of Mental Sciences over a 24-month period (DiClemente et al., 1994). Subjects from this 1994 sample had a mean age of 34 years (ranging from 18 to 62). The majority of subjects were white (81.5%), and had about 12 years of education (ranging from 4 to 21). Approximately one-third of this sample was married, and 43% were separated or divorced. Thus unlike CRC members, who are in recovery, this sample consists of people applying for treatment. They are also older and more likely to be married and were probably not in college. To facilitate this comparison, a difference score (Cohen's D) was computed by subtracting the DiClemente et al. (1994) sample means from the CRC sample means and then dividing by the average of the two standard deviations. Reflecting their recovery status, CRC members seem less tempted to drink in general, reporting less temptation to drink on 18 of the 19 items. The scores for the other item were identical. The differences were the most noticeable on the Physical/Other Concerns subscale where CRC members reported scores between 1.04 and 1.75 standard deviations lower than scores for the clinical sample. As stated previously, it is possible that the low score of the CRC sample on this subscale were due to the younger age of CRC members.

The smallest differences were found on the negative affect scale. As mentioned earlier, for this young group of recovering addicts, dealing with negative affect appears to be significantly more difficult than dealing with other triggers to use. For this subscale, their scores reflect being more tempted to drink when experiencing negative affect.

Alcohol Abstinence Self-Efficacy Summary. These results indicate that on average, CRC members reported being "not very tempted" to drink across a range of nineteen potential alcohol-use trigger situations. In comparison with the sample respondents in DiClemente et al. (1994) study, CRC members reported lower scores on 18 of the 19 items used in this study. Respondents from the CRC were more tempted to drink when experiencing negative affect as opposed to physical pain, withdrawals/cravings, or social situations. There were no statistically significant differences when examining AASE subscale mean scores by biological sex. However, length of recovery items indicate that respondents who have been in drug abuse recovery for less than 6 months are significantly more tempted to drink in all four of the contexts assessed by the AASE subscales than respondents who reported longer lengths of drug abuse recovery. That significant differences were found for length of recovery, but not for time in the community, may reflect the fact that during data collection, many new members were joining, but not all of these new members arrived with the same levels of recovery stability—as those whose time in recovery was shorter appear to be more at risk.

Stage of Change (URICA)

Table 5.5 presents information on the levels of action and maintenance behavior among CRC members as well as similar data from three comparison samples.

Table 5.5 University of Rhode Island Change Assessment (URICA) scores

Sample	n	M	SD	Male	Female	$\acute{a}$
Action scale						
TTU CRC	72	3.92	0.68	3.97	3.83	0.83
Incarcerated adolescent boys (Cohen et al., 2005)	131	3.51	0.84			
Adolescent inpatients (Greenstein et al., 1999)	89	3.66	0.75			
Adult outpatients (McConnaughy et al., 1989)	327	3.47	0.79			
Maintenance scale						
TTU CRC	71	3.36	0.67	3.41	3.24	0.71
Incarcerated adolescent boys (Cohen et al., 2005)	131	2.88	0.80			
Adolescent inpatients (Greenstein et al., 1999)	89	3.28	0.75			
Adult outpatients (McConnaughy et al., 1989)	327	3.21	0.79			

Comparison data were from incarcerated adolescent males (Cohen et al., 2005), adolescents receiving psychiatric care (Greenstein, Franklin, & McGuffin, 1999), and adult outpatients (McConnaughy, DiClemente, Prochaska, & Velicer, 1989). The top half of the table presents action scores; maintenance scores are below. An initial observation about for CRC member's data is that the mean score for the "action" subscale ($M = 3.92$) was higher than the mean score for the "maintenance" subscale ($M = 3.36$). This is the same pattern observed for each comparison sample (see Table 5.5).

It should also be noted that the CRC scores appear somewhat higher than those of the comparison samples. This pattern was especially marked for the Action subscale, for which the CRC mean (3.92) was approximately half a standard deviation higher than those of the comparison samples (3.51, 3.66, and 3.47, respectively). The Maintenance mean of the CRC sample was also higher than comparison samples, but to less of a degree.

Reflecting upon the 12-step culture around which this community is organized may shed some light on members' responses. According to a 12-step perspective, one never is cured of an addiction. Instead, the addict—who is always an addict— can hold addiction at bay by working the 12 steps. Considering this perspective, it would seem that CRC members are sustaining their recoveries by actively working their program. Consonant with this perspective is the finding that the CRC members while reporting somewhat higher maintenance scores than the comparison samples, reported substantially higher (0.55 of a SD greater) action scores than any of the comparison samples. Taken together, these findings are consistent with a picture of a community that is very devoted to sustaining recovery a fashion consistent with 12-step principles. As a group, they appear to be focusing on actively working their program rather than progressing to a point where they think they have defeated their problem and need only focus on maintenance behaviors. This might indicate that in terms of DiClemente and Prochaska's (1982, 1985) stages of change, CRC members (as most of the other comparison samples) are generally more entrenched in *actions* of behavioral coping and other change process activities ($M = 3.92$) than they are in *maintenance* ($M = 3.36$), which is the continued action to reinforce and establish the new behavior change into their lifestyle (DiClemente & Hughes, 1990; Prochaska & DiClemente, 1986a, 1986b). Secondly, the mean scores on these subscales suggest respondents generally "agree" with statements regarding action and CRC members' responses are between "undecided" and "agree" when responding to statements regarding maintenance.

Biological sex. Table 5.5 also presents the means for the URICA subscales by biological sex. Compared with females, males reported marginally higher mean scores on both subscales, but differences were not significant.

Length of drug abuse or drug dependency recovery. Table 5.6 presents mean scores for the URICA subscales by respondents' length of recovery. Upon a visual inspection of the table means, two patterns are evident. First, despite their being in treatment most recently, the group reporting six or fewer months since treatment reported the lowest levels of action and the highest levels of maintenance. Statistical analyses revealed that these differences were not significant (likely due to the small sample size of this group). However, when the pattern reported by this group is compared with other groups, especially to those in the 5+ years of recovery group, a clear difference in the relative focus on action vs. maintenance is observed. Members early in recovery reported nearly equal amounts of action and maintenance behaviors. In contrast, members with 5+ years of recovery reported substantially higher action than maintenance scores. Perhaps the responses of those with longer recoveries reflect this internalization of 12-step principles. Specifically that recovery is something that one actively "works" rather than waiting around for being surprised by ongoing challenges to their recoveries.

Table 5.6 University of Rhode Island Change Assessment (URICA) scores by length of recovery

URICA	0–6 months	7–24 months	2–5 years	5+ years
Action scale	3.60 (0.91)	4.00 (0.44)	3.93 (0.91)	3.74 (0.49)
Maintenance scale	3.68 (0.85)	3.39 (0.49)	3.50 (0.70)	2.78 (0.79)
	$n = 5$	$n = 24$	$n = 26$	$n = 11$

Because of the sizes of the groups being compared, formal significance tests found little. The only significant difference was between the maintenance scores of those members who had been in recovery between 7 and 24 months ($m = 3.39$) and those with 5+ years ($m = 2.78$).

Discussion

This chapter looked at three discrete but related phenomena: The temptations to use substances faced by CRC members in an abstinence-hostile collegiate environment, the tactics they use to resist these temptations, and the stage of recovery at which they consider themselves.

Regarding tactics, findings from the analyses of the APOC subscales indicate that instead of leaning primarily on physical interventions such as medications to assist with their recovery maintenance, CRC members rely more often on helping relationships, including the social support provided both formally and informally by the CSAR. This finding supports Rogers's (1951) longstanding theory of helping relationships and also the claim of Anthony, Rogers, and Farkas (2003) that relational factors are more important than any other technique or treatment for recovery maintenance. Social support appears to provide a buffer or protection from stressful events or pathogenic influences (Cohen & Wills, 1985).

Regarding temptations, results from the AASE subscales suggest that CRC members are most susceptible to temptations to drink when experiencing negative affect. Perhaps these respondents learned to rely on drugs and alcohol as a means of coping with daily stressors before they developed other, more positive means of coping to deal with challenges in relationships and education. These stressors are an unavoidable part of any adult life and CRC members must learn to cope with negative affect if they are to be successful in maintaining long-term recovery.

Action vs. Maintenance

One of the most interesting set of results from the present study came from analysis of the URICA, which traces stages of change in dealing with a problem such as substance addiction. Two main findings should be highlighted. The first is that the CRC sample appeared to identify more with the action than the maintenance stage. The second is that this pattern was particularly pronounced among students who had been in recovery the longest.

As noted in the Results, the first finding can easily be understood within the context of the 12-step culture around which the community is organized. Results from the URICA subscales indicate that CRC members despite having relatively stable recoveries are more involved in *actions* of behavioral coping than they are in *maintenance* behaviors. Moreover, more time in recovery does not correspond to more maintenance, but relatively less. Thus, members of this recovery community do not pass through the action stage into the maintenance stage, but stay focused on action behaviors.

Consistent with the notion that recovery is a process, rather than a task that can be completed, this pattern suggested that CRC members considered themselves to be "recovering," rather than "recovered" but tempted to backslide. Thus, they are more likely to endorse Action items such as "At times my problem is difficult, but I am working on it" than Maintenance items such as "I thought once I had resolved the problem I would be free of it, but sometimes I still find myself struggling with it," or "It worries me that I might slip back on a problem I have already changed, so I am here to seek help" (CPRC, 2003). Arguably, each of the items on the Maintenance scale represents a type of cognitive distortion: The illusion that recovery was, at some point, complete. Perhaps members of a recovery community that is organized by 12-step principles should not progress beyond a focus on action to a focus on maintenance, at least not in the way maintenance is defined by Prochaska and DiClemente (1986a). Individuals treating recovery as a process have, in essence, asserted day-to-day control over their addictions. Consistent with AA principles, they have recognized addiction as a powerful force, and they only way to deal with it is to assert their own will, their own agency, on a continuous basis (see Maruna, 2001). Moreover, affiliation with AA or NA does not cure addiction; rather, active addiction and the self-centeredness that underlies it are held at bay by actively practicing 12-step principles (Humphreys, 2004). Their 12-step recovery has empowered them to fight back, even as, at the same time, they know that the foe will never be wholly vanquished (Yeh, Che, Lee, & Horng, 2008).

The illusion the recovery can be complete, however, appears to be more attractive to the CRC members who had been in treatment or recovery for the shortest periods. The second finding, that maintenance diminished in importance relative to action as time in recovery increased, suggests a different stage theory: After the precontemplation and contemplation stages, their initial action phase, comprising intensive treatment, led to complacency, which was disturbed only by the realization, consistent with the AA principle of continuous self-inventory, that recovery was not in fact complete but needed to be constantly worked. Only after the complacency ends and disequilibrium sets in can the mature "maintaining through action" stage begin. An examination of the Maintenance items of the URICA reveals that they actually indicate that the individual has recognized the dissonance between the idea that s/he'd taken care of the problem and the realization that s/he could use a little more help, a little more work. In contrast, many of the Action items reflect the continuing nature, and continuing challenges, of recovery (e.g., "I am really working hard to change"), although some (e.g., "I have started working on my problems but I would like help") are oriented toward the beginning of recovery. In the future, an instrument could be developed that would enable a test of this refined stage model that incorporates these cognitive shifts: precontemplation, contemplation, initial action, complacency, disequilibrium, and maintenance through continuing action—i.e., "recovery." As Prochaska and DiClemente (1982) acknowledge, individuals might enter and exit recovery several times during their lives. The proposed stage model suggests that it is likely that both complacency and disequilibrium would be risk factors for relapse, but for very different reasons. Identification of these stages would allow for interventions to be more precisely targeted.

Conclusions

This chapter examined the strategies that members use to maintain their sobriety and the situations that challenge this sobriety. Taken as a whole, the findings in this chapter provide professionals and researchers with some insight into how young adults in a collegiate recovery environment manage temptations and utilize tactics to maintain recovery in an abstinence-hostile environment. These findings are consistent with conclusions of other chapters regarding the importance of social support young adults in recovery, and comport with the 12-step model that sees addiction, though incurable, as something that can be handled. The highlights are that community members rely heavily on helping relationships. This reliance is consistent with the design of the Collegiate Recovery Community, which the CSAR has grown is size to provide ample opportunities for it members to form supportive friendships with young adults who share histories of abuse and current commitments to recovery. Members' susceptibility to negative mood is not surprising. However, these findings can help CSAR staff as well as others who work with recovering young adults, such as those working to establish new collegiate recovery programs, be mindful of the difficulty that negative mood presents for this population. Finding that members are more focused on action stage than the maintenance stage of change, and that over time in the community members focus on action suggests that the protective context the CRC provides is not leading members to a false and dangerous sense of complacency. As 12 steppers know, the price of liberty, at least from drugs, is eternal vigilance.

References

Annis, H. M., & Martin, G. (1985). *The drug-taking confidence questionnaire*. Toronto, Ontario, Canada: Addiction Research Foundation of Ontario.

Anthony, W., Rogers, E. S., & Farkas, M. (2003). Research on evidence-based practices: Future directions in an era of recovery. *Community Mental Health Journal, 39*, 101–114.

Baumeister, R. F., Smart, L., & Boden, J. M. (1996). Relation of threatened egotism to violence and aggression: The dark side of high self-esteem. *Psychological Review, 103*, 5–33.

Bogenschutz, M. P., Tonigan, S., & Miller, W. P. (2006). Examining the effects of alcoholism typology and AA attendance on self-efficacy as a mechanism of change. *Journal of Studies on Alcohol, 67*, 562–567.

Bruning, J. L., & Kintz, B. L. (1987). *Computational handbook of statistics*. Glenview, Illinois: Scott Foresman & Co.

Callaghan, R. C., Hathaway, A., Cunningham, J. A., Vettese, L. C., Wyatt, S., & Taylor, L. (2005). Does stage-of-change predict dropout in a culturally diverse sample of adolescents admitted to inpatient substance-abuse treatment? A test of the Transtheoretical Model. *Addictive Behaviors, 30*, 1834–1847.

Cancer Prevention Research Center (2003). *Alcohol: Processes of change*. http://www.uri.edu/research/cprc/Measures/Alcohol06.htm.

Cohen, P. J., Glaser, B. A., Calhoun, G. B., Bradshaw, C. P., & Petrocelli, J. V. (2005). Examining readiness for change: A preliminary evaluation of the University of Rhode Island Change Assessment with incarcerated adolescents. *Measurement and Evaluation in Counseling and Development, 38*, 45–62.

Cohen, S., & Wills, T. A. (1985). Stress, social support and the buffering hypothesis. *Psychological Bulletin, 95*, 310–357.

Demmel, R., Nicolal, J., & Jenko, D. M. (2006). Self-efficacy and alcohol relapse: Concurrent validity of confidence measures, self-other discrepancies, and prediction of treatment outcome. *Journal of Studies on Alcohol, 67*, 637–641.

DiClemente, C., Carbonari, J., Montgomery, R., & Hughes, S. (1994). The alcohol abstinence self-efficacy scale. *Journal of Studies on Alcohol, 55*, 141–148.

DiClemente, C. C., & Hughes, S. O. (1990). Stages of change profiles in outpatient alcoholism treatment. *Journal of Substance Abuse, 2*, 217–235.

DiClemente, C. C., & Prochaska, J. O. (1982). Self-change and therapy change of smoking behavior: A comparison of processes of change in cessation and maintenance. *Addictive Behaviors*, *7*, 133–142.

DiClemente, C. C., & Prochaska, J. O. (1985). Processes and stages of self-change: Coping and competence in smoking behavior change. In S. Shiffman & T. A. Wills (Eds.), *Coping behavior and drug use*. San Diego, CA: Academic.

Greenstein, D. K., Franklin, M. E., & McGuffin, P. (1999). Measuring motivation to change: An examination of the University of Rhode Island Change Assessment questionnaire (URICA) in an adolescent sample. *Psychotherapy*, *36*, 47–55.

Henderson, M. J., Saules, K. K., & Galen, L. W. (2004). The predictive validity of the University of Rhode Island Change Assessment Questionnaire in a heroin-addicted polysubstance use sample. *Psychology of Addictive Behaviors*, *18*, 106–112.

Humphreys, K. (2004). *Circles of recovery: Self-help organizations for addictions*. Cambridge, UK: Cambridge University Press.

Maruna, S. (2001). *Making good: How ex-convicts reform and rebuild their lives*. Washington, DC: American Psychological Association.

McConnaughy, E. A., DiClemente, C. C., Prochaska, J. O., & Velicer, W. F. (1989). Stages of change in psychotherapy: A follow-up report. *Psychotherapy*, *26*, 494–503.

McConnaughy, E. A., Prochaska, J. O., & Velicer, W. F. (1983). Stages of change in psychotherapy: Measurement and sample profiles. *Psychotherapy: Theory, Research, & Practice*, *20*, 368–375.

National Institute on Alcohol Abuse and Alcoholism (2000). *University of Rhode Island change assessment scale (URICA)*. NIAAA Publications. http://www.niaaa.nih.gov/publications/urica.htm.

Prochaska, J. O., & DiClemente, C. C. (1982). Transtheoretical therapy: Toward a more integrative model of change. *Psychotherapy: Theory, Research, & Practice*, *19*, 276–288.

Prochaska, J. O., & DiClemente, C. C. (1986a). Toward a comprehensive model of change. In W. R. Miller & N. Heather (Eds.), *Treating addictive behaviors* (pp. 3–27). New York: Plenum.

Prochaska, J. O., & DiClemente, C. C. (1986b). The transtheoretical approach: Towards a systematic eclectic framework. In J. C. Norcross (Ed.), *Handbook of eclectic psychotherapy*. New York: Brunner/Mazel.

Rogers, C. R. (1951). *Client-centered therapy*. Boston, MA: Houghton Mifflin.

Sklar, S. M., Annis, H. M., & Turner, N. E. (1999). Group comparisons of coping self-efficacy between alcohol and cocaine abusers seeking treatment. *Psychology of Addictive Behaviors*, *13*, 122–133.

Sutton, S. (2001). Back to the drawing board? A review of applications of the transtheoretical model to substance use. *Addiction*, *96*, 175–186.

Yeh, M., Che, H., Lee, L., & Horng, F. (2008). An empowerment process: Successful recovery from alcohol dependence. *Journal of Clinical Nursing*, *17*, 921–929.

Chapter 6
Daily Lives of Young Adult Members of a Collegiate Recovery Community

H. Harrington Cleveland and Allison Groenendyk

The Collegiate Recovery Community(CRC) at Texas Tech University (TTU) provides both a safe haven for those in recovery to maintain their abstinence and a social environment that nurtures the personal development. To provide information of how the recovery community functions we collected information on members' daily experiences using end-of-day palm pilot data collections. The goal of these data collections was to assess the daily lives of community members as they maintain their recovery status "one day at a time." The resulting data provide insight into what it means to be part of the CRC at TTU. Using these data, this chapter details the daily social experiences connecting individual members of the community to different parts of their social worlds, which while strongly influenced by other members of the community are also made up of people in recovery who are not members of the Collegiate Recovery Community and college students who are not in recovery. Ideally, these social experiences provide social support for continued abstinence while allowing members to have developmentally appropriate social experiences that will help them build stronger selves.

The Value of Daily Diary Data Collections

In order investigate the how the social, as well as individual, experiences of members support or challenge their abstinence, we collected data using daily dairy data collection methods. By capturing life as it is lived, diary methods, unlike single administration correlational or long-term panel designs, use daily, or more frequent, data collections to assess and examine both daily and across day patterns of emotional and psychological states, such as substance use cravings and negative moods, and social support experiences, such as conversations with friends (Bolger, Davis, & Rafaeli, 2003). Using multilevel models, such data can be used to rule out

H.H. Cleveland (✉)
The Pennsylvania State University, University Park, PA, USA
e-mail: cleveland@psu.edu

H.H. Cleveland et al. (eds.), *Substance Abuse Recovery in College*, Advancing
Responsible Adolescent Development, DOI 10.1007/978-1-4419-1767-6_6,
© Springer Science+Business Media, LLC 2010

person-level third-variable influences, such as personality traits (Bolger, DeLongis, Kessler, & Schilling, 1989), on associations between within and between day phenomena. However, in addition to this increasingly conventional application is their ability to create high-quality reports of daily activities that avoid the substantial measurement bias associated with retrospective reporting of social events (Bolger et al., 2003). Applied to the lives of CRC community members this method provides detailed end-of-day reports of individual days social and individual behaviors that are both more accurate person-level information than data drawn from single administration data collections, but also provide detailed information about within-person variation in social and individual experiences. Such data have been used extensively in the fields of stress research, where for example they have been used to investigate the effects of interpersonal tensions (Almeida, 2005), as well as the examination of the within-day links between stressors and alcohol use among regular (Armeli, Carney, Tennen, Affleck, & O'Neal, 2000) and problem drinkers (Mohr et al., 2001).

Social Contact: The Substrate of Abstinence Support

For this study, we use these methods to investigate the social support for abstinence that CRC members experience as part of the TTU Collegiate Recovery Community. Prior research has consistently concluded that the social support that affiliates receive from other group members is one of the primary reasons that AA affiliation protects abstinence (Longabaugh & Beattie, 1986; Beattie & Longabaugh, 1997). This social support appears to buffer the effects of social influences and triggers that may otherwise challenge recovery (Longabaugh, Wirtz, Zweben, & Stout, 1998) and mediates a substantial portion of the association between 12-step affiliation and abstinence likelihood (Humphreys, Mankowski, Moos, & Finney, 1999). The new abstaining friends that 12-step affiliated gain by group membership appear to aid abstinence whether they replace old substance using friends (Humphreys & Noke, 1997) or simply provide insulation against the influence of these drinking friends (Bond, Kaskutas, & Weisner, 2003). For this reason, our diary data collection focused on respondents' social experiences, focusing our questions on the frequency, duration, and nature of social contact with abstinence and nonabstinent friends. Because we were particularly interested in the role the CSAR drop-in-center and the CRC itself played in the daily lives of CRC members we used separate sets of questions to collect information about social contact with members of the Collegiate Recovery Community at and away from the drop-in-center, 12-step people who are not affiliated with the Collegiate Recovery Community and nonrecovery friends. In addition, we present data on daily interactions with family members, self-improvement behaviors, and smoking behaviors.

Methods

Procedures. Using daily data collection methods we gathered information on the daily social support and individual experiences that support and threaten abstinence from 55 members of the Collegiate Recovery Community. Participants were recruited during the community's weekly organizational meetings. During recruitment, the nature of the study, including that it was a diary study that involved baseline questionnaires and a minimum of 3 weeks of end-of-day Palm Pilot data entries, was explained to community members. It was also explained that participation was voluntary, that data were confidential but not anonymous, and that each participant would be compensated with $50. Community members who were willing to participate were assigned to four different data collection flights, one in the fall of 2004, two in the spring of 2005, and one in the fall of 2005.

Each data collection flight began with a baseline questionnaire and instructions on how to use a palm pilot to make end-of-day data entries. Following completion of the baseline questionnaire and practicing a data entry with the Palm Pilot, participants were instructed to begin end-of-day data collections that evening, and continue data entry over the weekend. After the first weekend, participants brought in their Palm Pilot for "Hot Syncing" (i.e., downloading). At this time, research staff transferred participants' first few days of data from their Palm Pilots to the project computer. This meeting allowed staff to ensure that data were being correctly saved, entered daily (examined with time stamps on each data entry), and that the Palm Pilots were being properly charged. It also provided a chance for staff to answer any participant questions.

The data collection program used for daily data entries recorded the start time and end time of each data collection. This information was used to examine compliance with single-end-of-day daily data entry protocol. Of the 60 participants who began the four flights, 55 completed the study. In spite of filling out the baseline, three participants failed to make daily data entries. Time stamps for one other participant's daily data entries revealed multiple data entries on the same days and brief durations—less than 4 min per entry—for data entries. A final participant filled out daily entries, but did not provide baseline information. Data entries for these five participants were dropped from the data set. The remaining 55 participants made between 15 and 33 data entries, totaling 1,319 daily entries for 23.7 days of data entries on average. Despite this substantial between-person range, nearly ninety percent of respondents (50) provided between 19 and 29 days of data. The three providing less than 19 daily entries provided 17, 15, and 15 respectively. The two providing more than 29 days provided 32 and 33 days each.

Participants. The analysis sample was made up of 39 males (71%) and 16 females (29%). Their average age was 22.6 ($SD = 5.7$). Ethnically, the sample, like the community it was drawn from, was homogenous. All but one of the 55 respondents chose "white, non-Hispanic" as their ethnic/racial background. One individual chose "American Indian/Other." In part, this racial/ethnic homogeneity reflects the enrollment of the university in which the recovery community is nested. However, it may also reflect the race/ethnicity of those young people with addictions who have the family financial resources to both receive intensive treatment for their addictions and attend college (See Cleveland et al., 2007).

Results

Social Contact: The Substrate of Abstinence Support

The most information we collected was a measure of the number of community members each respondent at least said "hi" to and how many they talked to for at least a few minutes that day. The maximum allowed response for both items was 50 people. Respondents' average daily contact was 7.2 ($SD = 8.1$) community members that they said hi to and 4.7 ($SD = 4.9$) that they talked to for at least a few minutes. There was considerable variation between respondents on these social contact measures. For example, on the high end of social contact 6 of the 55 respondents reported saying hi to an average of more than 15 other community members and 8 respondents averaged talking to over 7 other community members per day. On the low end, 15 respondents reported saying "hi" to fewer than 5 other members a day and 8 respondents "talked" to less than 2 members a day. This range indicates that the community includes members who have a great deal of social contact with other members, as well as members whose community social contact much is more limited. Social contact also varied between days. For example, on 14% and 16% of days there was no "saying hello" or talking to other community members.

Social Exchanges at the Community Drop-In Center

To collect detailed information about respondents' social experiences with community members we asked blocks of questions about their activities and conversations with community members, both while at the drop-in-center and outside of the center. Because it is a unique aspect of the CRC at TTU, we asked very specific questions about the social interactions that occur at the drop-in-center. Responses indicated that 37% of days (489 out of a possible 1,318) included time spent at the drop-in-center. Again, there were substantial differences among respondents: Seven people stopped by the drop-in-center on 70% of days or more and 12 people stopping by on only 20% of days or less. In fact, 2 respondents did not report ever stopping by the drop-in-center during the duration of their data entry period.

Most visits to the drop-in-center were not brief. Only 7% and 4% of visits were just stopping by to say "hi" or for a just a few minutes and another 17% of visits were between 5 and 15 min long. More commonly, 72% total, visits were longer, 20% between 15 and 30 min, 22% between 30 and 60 min, and 19% between 1 and 2 h. A final 10% were longer than 2 h.

At the drop-in-center people talked about various topics. But nearly always (89%; 433 of 489 visits) their visits included just hanging out and talking. In terms of substantive topics, it was most common to talk about school/academic issues (55%). Recent (27%) and future social events (26%) were also commonly discussed. Money issues (10%), roommate (7%) and family issues (8%) arose less frequently. Past treatment and substance use experiences came up, but only for 7% and 8% of the visits.

On 130 of the 489 visits to the drop-in-center, respondents reported they witnessed someone giving advice or sharing an experience to help another person. The advice or shared- story was as likely to be from a staff member (62%) as a community friend (68%), such as a member with a history of both alcohol and drug use, an alcohol-only history (21%), a drug-only history (24%), or an eating disorder member (15%). While the frequencies of advice from members with different addictive histories approximately reflect their percentages in the entire community, it is notable that CSAR staff members play such an active role in giving advice and sharing stories of their pasts. That they can play this role may reflect the fact that several of the staff members are in recovery themselves. Topically, "advice" was more likely to be about academics (53%) or college social life (58%) than about dealing with stress (35%), family issues (24%), or roommates (8%). Given where these conversations occurred, it should not be surprising that 74% of the advice across these topics were discussed in terms of recovery. Also reflecting the helping nature of this environment, respondents reported that on 31% of their visits they witnessed someone else offer to help or express concern for another person.

Outside of Center Contact with Community Members

As explained in other chapters in this volume, it is a principle of the CSAR is that the primary social support benefits of community membership comes other community members, rather than from staff at the drop-in-center. To determine the extent that members' community social support is derived from out of center contact with other community members, as well as the relative quantity and type that they are receiving from different aspects of their social support network (i.e., community friends, noncommunity 12-step friends, and "normie" friends), end-of-day data collections captured detailed information on participants' social contact. As expected, participants reported spending substantial amounts of social time with other members of the Collegiate Recovery Community (see Table 6.1). Specifically, respondents indicated that they spent social time or talked to a community friend outside of the center on 72% (950/1317) of study days. On these 950 days the most common interactions with other community members were casual talk (699) and phone calls (482). Not all talk was light-hearted, however. As on 21% of these days (201 of 950) respondents indicated that their social time with other community friends included "heavy emotional" talk. Although phone calls and casual talk were the most common activities

Table 6.1 Frequency of activities performed with friends

Activity	CRC	Local 12-step	"Normies"	Total
Totals	949	467	586	2,002
Phone call	482	177	482	1,141
Casual talk	699	324	388	1,411
Heavy talk	201	95	49	345
Lunch	250	40	74	364
Dinner	430	91	114	635
Sports/workout	57	25	50	132
Dry party	86	20	11	117
Went to bar/club	53	12	65	130
Studied	67	15	62	144
TV/DVD	348	59	77	832
Went to movies	27	5	10	42
Shopping	48	10	10	68

with other community members, respondents did not have substantially different odds of doing these activities with CSAR members as they did with noncommunity 12-step people or with nonrecovering friends "normies" (Table 6.2). Respondents did, however, have 2.94 greater odds of reporting a heavy emotional talk with other community members than with normies.

Table 6.2 Odds ratios comparing frequency of activities between groups

	CRC: 12-step	CRC: normies	12 step: normies	12-step: CRC	Normies: 12-step	Normies: CRC
Phone call	1.69	0.22	0.13	0.59	7.59	4.49
Casual talk	1.23	1.43	1.16	0.81	0.86	0.70
Heavy talk	1.05	2.94	2.80	0.95	0.36	0.34
Lunch	3.82	2.47	0.65	0.26	1.54	0.40
Dinner	3.42	3.43	1.00	0.29	1.00	0.29
Sports/workout	1.13	0.69	0.61	0.89	1.65	1.46
Dry party	2.23	5.21	2.34	0.45	0.43	0.19
Went to bar/club	2.24	0.47	0.21	0.45	4.73	2.11
Studied	2.29	0.64	0.28	0.44	3.57	1.56
TV/DVD	4.00	3.83	0.96	0.25	1.05	0.26
Went to movies	2.71	1.69	0.62	0.37	1.60	0.59
Shopping	2.43	3.07	1.26	0.41	0.79	0.33

It was common for community members to eat together, 251 times for lunch and 432 times for dinner of the 950 days (Table 6.1). The higher frequency for dinner likely reflects many members being housemates with each other. As noted in Chapter 2 , every effort is made to match members of the community with other members with whom they can share a house or apartment. Being housemates with other community members provide them contact with their abstinence-supportive social network while at home in the evenings. While at their own homes or perhaps at the residence of other community members, it seems that the most common activity was watching TV and DVDs with other community members. This activity was reported on 348 (37%) of the 950 days that respondents spent social time with community members outside of the center. They also report going to parties while with community friends. When with community members, respondents were more likely to go to "dry" parties (86 times) than parties or bars with substance using others (53 times).

Odds ratios (Table 6.2) were used to more formally capture the degree to which these more common activities were more likely with community members than with other aspects of their social networks relative to the total number of days that they spent with these types of friends. Take for example having lunch, even considering their higher number of days with community members respondents had 3.82 and 3.42 greater odds, respectively, of going to lunch with them than with local 12-steppers or with normies. They also had greater odds of eating dinner with community members than with local 12-steppers or with normies (odds =3.42 and 3.43, respectively). Further, respondents had greater odds of watching TV or DVD's with community members, than with either local 12-steppers (odds = 4.00) or normies (odds = 3.83). Additionally, respondents had greater odds of attending dry parties with community members than with 12-steppers (odds = 2.23), but especially than with normies (odds = 5.21).

When with community members, participants were most likely to talk about college social life (85%; Table 6.3). This was followed by academics (58%), dealing with stress (34%), family issues (28%), and roommates (21%). Conversations about college social life and roommates were both more relatively common in this setting than at the drop-in-center. However, it was less common, only 50% of the time compared to over 74% at the drop-in-center, that these topics would be discussed in terms of recovery. This difference may reflect both the characteristics of community members who spent more time at the center and the effect of being at home spending time with friends rather than at the center.

Table 6.3 Frequency of conversation topics performed with friends

Topics	CSAR	Local 12-step	"Normies"	Total
Totals	950	468	591	2,009
Academics	550	191	287	1,028
College/social life	805	355	467	1,627
Family issues	262	108	113	483
Roommate issues	195	55	51	301
Dealing with stress	319	151	116	586

Despite these very common conversation topics, odds ratios suggest that there was not much difference in topics discussed with community members as compared to conversation topics with noncommunity 12-steppers and normies (Table 6.4). Odds ratios did show, however, that respondents had 2.73 greater odds of talking

Table 6.4 Odds ratios comparing frequency of conversation topics between groups

	CRC: 12-step	CRC: normies	12 step: normies	12-step: CRC	Normies: 12-step	Normies: CRC
Academics	1.99	1.46	0.73	0.50	1.37	0.69
College/social life	1.77	1.47	0.83	0.57	1.20	0.68
Family issues	1.27	1.61	1.27	0.79	0.79	0.62
Roommate issues	1.94	2.73	1.41	0.52	0.71	0.37
Dealing with stress	1.06	2.07	1.95	0.94	0.51	0.48

about roommate issues with other community members than with normies and 2.07 greater odds of discussing ways to deal with stress with community members than with normies.

Not only was spending social time with recovery community members a common activity in terms of the percentage of days, the number of hours each day spent with this part of their social network was quite substantial. In fact, most days when out of center social time with community members was reported the amount of time with these friends was 2 h or more. Specifically, 2–3 h was reported of 26% and 4 h of more on 56% of days. Time spent on the remaining days with out of center social time was distributed between 1 and 2 h (10%), a ½ h (5%), and a few minutes (4%). This distribution makes it clear that community members do not have to come by the community's drop-in-center to have contact with the protective community that it provides. Moreover, they appear to actually get most of their community contact outside the drop-in-center.

Social Contact with Noncommunity 12-Step People

Although social contact with 12-step affiliates who were not part of the Collegiate Recovery Community was less frequent than with members of the community, such contact occurred on over a third (467; 36%) of the study days (Table 6.1). The part of participants' social network includes other college students who were in recovery, but not part of the center; people who were in recovery and who did not attend the university, including those affiliated with off campus meetings and 12-step friends from respondents' hometown 12-step programs (if they were not part of the CRC). This social contact could also include sponsor contact, but specific questions about sponsor contact were also included (reported below). Just like time with community friends, the most common social activities with noncommunity friends were casual talk (324 days; 69%) and phone calls (117 days; 25%). Also similar to out of center social contact with community members, social contact with this part of their social network included "heavy emotional" talk about one fifth (96 days; 21%) of the 467 days on which it occurred.

Despite the higher relative frequency of contact with these individuals than normies, odds ratios show that respondents were no more likely to talk on the phone or have casual talk with local 12-step individuals than with normies (Table 6.2). Odds ratios do suggest, however, that respondents had 2.80 greater odds of having heavy emotional conversation with local 12-steppers than with normies. This highlights that respondents were more likely to open up to individuals with similar experiences than with nonrecovering friends.

Relatively infrequent behaviors with noncommunity 12-steppers were having lunch (40 days; 9%) or dinner (90 days; 19%; Table 6.1). When with these noncommunity members, respondents were comparatively more likely to go to "dry" parties (20 times; 4%), than go to "wet" parties (12 times; 3%). Respondents only reported watching TV and DVDs with their noncommunity recovery friends on 59 days, which was only 13% of the days spent with noncommunity recovery friends. Thus, compared to the time they spend with their community friends, it seems respondents' social time with noncommunity recovery friends is different both in terms of amount and in how it is spent. They seem to spend a lot of time, nearly every day and for several hours a day (watching TV, etc.), with community friends. In contrast, they spend less time with noncommunity 12-steppers.

Despite these notable differences, odds ratios suggest that respondents are not more relatively likely to do many activities with local 12-steppers than with community members or normies (Table 6.2). Respondents, however, did report a 2.34 greater odds of attending a dry party with a local 12-stepper than they do with normies. This likely reflects the recovering status of both members of the CRC and noncommunity recovering friends such that respondents avoid risky situations when with this population.

Perhaps because many of these 12-step friends are drawn from off campus meetings, compared to time with community members, talks with them were somewhat less likely to discuss academics (41%), college social life (76%), and roommate issues (12%; Table 6.3). However, they were similarly likely to discuss both family issues (23%) and dealing with stress (32%) with these friends as with their community friends. Just like talks with community friends, 50% of these topics were discussed in terms of recovery. Odds ratios, however, showed that few of these topics were much more or less likely with non community 12-steppers than with other groups. The exceptions perhaps being talking about "dealing with stress," which was 1.95 more likely to occur for this group than with normies and "talking about academics," which had half (0.5) the odds of happening with noncommunity vs. community 12-steppers.

Time Spent with People Not in Recovery

Of course, not all of community members' time is spent with friends who are also in recovery. Contact with these friends, who are often referred to as "normies" by many community members, was reported on 44% (586) of study days (Table 6.1). Just like for other parts of their social networks, the most common occurrence during time with these friends was casual talk (388 days, 66%) and phone calls (482; 82%).

However, heavy emotional talk was relatively rare. Such talk occurred on only 49 of the days (8%) spent with "normies," compared to such talk occurring on 21% of the days with social contact with community members and 20% of the days with noncommunity recovery friends.

Odds ratios demonstrate that respondents had much greater odds of talking on the phone with their normie friends than with either noncommunity recovering friends or community friends (odds = 4.49 and 7.59, respectively; Table 6.2). Unlike respondents' recovering friends who they were more like to see regularly at community and 12-step events, respondents keep in touch with their normie friends by phone.

These friends were also very unlikely to join respondents at a "dry" party, only 10 occasions (2%) during their time together (Table 6.1). However, 65 of the days (11%) they spent with these friends included time at a party or bar where others are using substances. Unlike community friends, respondents reported watching TV or DVDs with their normie friends on relatively few days (77; 13%). Additionally, respondents reported studying with their normie friends on 62 of the 586 days (11%).

Odds ratios support the conclusion that respondents have greater odds of going to a party or bar where there are others who are using substances than with 12-steppers or community friends (odds = 4.73 and 2.11, respectively; Table 6.2). Respondents also have 3.57 greater odds of studying with their normie friends than with noncommunity 12-steppers, which is likely because many of the noncommunity 12-step friends were not themselves in college.

In some ways, the relative occurrence of different topics during talks with the "normies" was similar to talks among community members (Table 6.3); for example, academics (49%), college social life (79%), and family issues (19%). However, the relative frequency of roommate issues (9%) being discussed was more similar to its occurrence among noncommunity recovery friends. Dealing with stress, however, was only a topic for 20% of these talks. Understandably, topics with normies were only discussed in terms of recovery 11% of the time, which was very different than the 50% of talks which were about recovery among both groups of recovery friends.

In sum, it seems that social contacts with nonrecovery friends are both less frequent than with community friends and less intense or emotionally close than time spent with either type of recovery friends (either within or outside the collegiate community). This difference may be due both to the amount of time members spend with community members and the intense nature of the common experiences that they share with both sets of their recovering friends. Without the same opportunities or natural connection with these nonrecovering friends, perhaps their friendships do not develop the same depth.

Given the particular risk that going to bars and parties where others were using substances would seem to present, we looked further into reports of these behaviors across respondents. Doing so we found that over the duration of the data collections, 23 of the 55 respondents reported going to a bar or "wet" party when they were with community friends. While the number of respondents going to bars with community members may seem high, the fact that this behavior occurs with community friends may reflect the high percentage of days (73%) and the amount of time each day that community members spend with each other. In comparison, this was only reported 10 times with noncommunity 12-step friends. This small number of respondents reporting going to a bar or wet party with noncommunity 12-step friends may be due to both the small percentage of days (36%) and that they may not be part of the college social scene. Thus, the lower number of respondents visiting bars and wet parties with them would be expected. Time spent with "normies" seems different. In spite of spending relatively few days with them (586 of 1,319 days, 44%) these friends end up going to bars and parties with just as many respondents (23 of 55 persons) as report going to bars and parties with the nearly ever-present community members, who they saw of 72% (949/1,319) of days. And unlike community members, these nonrecovery friends may be drinking in front of respondents. Thus, it does seem that time spent with "normies" carries with it an increased risk of exposure to social contexts that include drinking.

Family Social Contact

Perhaps reflecting the cell phone generation of current college students, respondents reported contact—either in person or by phone—with family members on 59% of days. Most commonly, this was with mothers (70%) or fathers (48%). But also included contact with a sister or brother, 14% and 20% of family social time days, respectively. Compared to the community friends, however, the amount of daily contact was very low—most reporting only a $\frac{1}{2}$ h (44%) or less (24%). We did not collect information on the topics participants discussed during these conversations.

Being Offered Alcohol

Although the majority of members' social lives seem to be spent with other members of the recovery community, the above information also demonstrates that members are exposed to social contexts, such as bars, clubs, and parties, where alcohol is present. In addition to their activities, the end-of-day questionnaire also asked them if they were offered alcohol that day. Over the 1,319 days, an offer of alcohol was reported on 93 days, which was 7% of days. On one hand, this represents only 1 day every 2 weeks on average. By this measure, the risk of being offered alcohol seems quite low. However, there was considerable variation across individuals. Approximately half ($n = 26$) of the respondents reported no offers of alcohol during the data collection period. And nine others report only one offer. Among more than a few respondents, however, receiving an offer of alcohol was quite common. Nine respondents (16.4% of the total) reported being offered alcohol on more than 5 days, with one of these reporting being offered alcohol on 10 of the 33 days they entered data. This suggests that within the Collegiate Recovery Community members are living substantially different lives; and although some exposure to alcohol should be expected for college students, it seems that nearly 1/5 of participants are still exposing themselves to contextual influences that would seem to increase their relapse risk.

It can be argued that part of the college experience is attending university/college events with other students, including sporting events. While these events do not occur everyday on a college campus, the heavy drinking atmosphere that surrounds some of them may present a substantial risk to people in recovery. It is hard to imagine a stronger message that drinking is normative than being surrounded by several thousand fellow students who are drinking that day. This party environment is most likely to occur at both football and basketball games. At these games a substantial portion of their fellow students will have consumed at least some alcohol and a smaller, but not insignificant, number will be inebriated. Inside this environment, students in recovery may become swept up in the party atmosphere and tempted to drink.

Based on their reports, respondents attended "sporting events" on 108 of the 1,319 days. As expected, the most popular events were football and basketball games, which made up 35 and 29% of the sporting events attended. Other sporting events attended, and the number of times they were reported in parentheses, were soccer (15), softball (9), baseball (5), and volleyball (3). On the one hand, it might be best for their abstinence if members of the community did not attend football and basketball games. On the other hand, part of these young men's and women's "recovery" includes participating in normative age appropriate activities. At a large university, such normative age appropriate activities often include attending football and basketball games. It is important to realize, however, that in other educational settings, such as smaller liberal arts schools, the social activities linked to heavy drinking may differ. Although there were no survey items addressing this, it is believed that members of the recovery community often attend these games together. Perhaps this is the best of both worlds then, being able to experience normative college life, but doing so surrounded by the protective influence of your recovering peers.

Working Their 12-Step Programs

Although both the Center for Study of Addiction and Recovery (CSAR) and the Collegiate Recovery Community (CRC) take a broad view of recovery, the community itself is organized around 12-step principles and culture. In fact, part of members' commitment to the community is a promise to attend at least two 12-step meetings a week. As a group, members have little problem meeting this commitment, reporting attending at least one 12-step meeting on 42% (550) of the 1,319 study days. Alcoholics Anonymous (AA) and Narcotics Anonymous (NA) meetings were the most commonly attended, with 278 and 150 occurrences, respectively. Nearly as common was attendance at the community's weekly Celebration of Recovery, with 132 occurrences. In addition to these meetings, members also reported attending Eating Disorder (9 occurrences) and Gambling Anonymous (6 occurrences) meetings. In addition to these meetings, "other" 12-step meetings (10) and non-12-step meetings (15) were also attended. Finally, respondents also reported attending ASAS meetings (Association of Students about Service) on 68 days. ASAS is the community's university recognized student run community governance organization. This meeting is held weekly during the hour preceding the Celebration of Recovery. Based on the number of times it was reported, it seems that about one half of the community attends these meetings.

All but two of our respondents reported currently having a 12-step sponsor. Those with sponsors report talking to them on 34% of days. Half of these days included in-person conversations, the other half only phone contact. When they did talk to sponsors, this was often about "general life issues" (66%) or just "saying hi" (42%). Less frequently talks were about an "abstinence specific" issue (23%) or working a specific step (21%). That most talks with sponsors were about general topics rather than being specifically about abstinence underscores that the importance of sponsors extends beyond providing specific tools to deal with challenges to recovery.

Beyond talking to their sponsors, respondents also report actively working their "programs" by applying 12-steps to their daily lives. They report applying at least one of the 12-steps on 77% of the study days. Of the different 12-steps, the most commonly applied were steps 1, 2, and 3, which were reported on 953, 729, and 802 days. These steps have been labeled the "surrender steps" (Tonigan, Ashcroft, & Miller, 1995). An example of a surrender step is "Admitted that we were powerless over alcohol/drugs—that our lives had become unmanageable" (Step 1). These steps were followed in frequency by Steps 10, 11, and 12, the "maintenance steps," which occurred 457, 465, and 397 times. An example of a maintenance step is "Continued to take personal inventory and when we were wrong promptly admitted it" (Step 10). In contrast to the frequent application of surrender and maintenance steps, "actions steps," which are Steps 4–9, were applied relatively infrequently—ranging from 15 days for Step 5 ("Admitted to God, to ourselves, and to another human being the exact nature of our wrongs"), which only occurred on 15 days, to 88 days for Steps 7 ("Humbly asked Him to remove our shortcomings"). In addition to helping capture the nature of how the 12-steps are applied on a daily basis to help maintain abstinence and build recovery, these data also demonstrate that the members of this community are very actively involved in the 12-step program.

Self-Improvement

Also reflecting the members' recovery status, respondents reported participating in self-improvement behaviors, such as reading 12-step literature, the Bible, going to church, etc., on 38% of days. The most common self-improvement behaviors participated in were reading Alcoholics Anonymous literature (229 days), doing 12-step meditations (107), reading the Bible (or other holy book; 96), and reading Narcotics Anonymous literature (64). Like the data on applying 12-steps to their daily lives, these data make it clear that in addition to enjoying the social support provided by the community, members are actively working their own recovery programs.

Notably less common than working their own programs was attending church, which was reported on only 12 of the total 1,319 days. Not only was church attendance very rare, but examining its distribution across respondents revealed that 8 of these 11 times were reported by only two respondents. Thus, while the community is generally organized around 12-step principles that may seem quasireligious, and members are actively "working the program," their church attendance does not suggest they are conventionally religious.

Smoking

As many observers of 12-step culture know, smoking is very common among people in recovery. Members of the Collegiate Recovery Community are no different. In fact, 41 of 55 respondents (75%) smoked a cigarette at least one day during the duration of the study. Among these "smokers" smoking was quite frequent. For the 1,002 total end-of-day reports entered by respondents who were "smokers," smoking was reported on 852 of them (85%). Not only did smoking respondents smoke frequently, they smoked a lot. On over 30% of smoking days, they report smoking either a full pack or more (31%) or between a half and a full pack (31%). Light smoking days were comparatively rare with 5–10 cigarettes being smoked on 22% of days and less than 5 being smoked on 16% of days. Consistent with their heavy use of tobacco, as well as their addictive histories, most smokers smoked early in the day. Nineteen percent of smoking days began with a cigarette within the first 5 min and 30% more with a cigarette within 30 min of waking. Days in which smoking began within the first hour accounted for another 21% of days. Only during 12% and 18% of smoking days was the first cigarette later in the morning or in the afternoon.

Discussion

Within these findings is a large amount of good news, some information that is difficult to interpret, and some bad news. Most of it, we think, is good news. First of all, while there is substantial between-person variation, the community seems to be defined by high frequency, close personal relationships, where community members seem to be nearly surrounded by abstinent others, both at and away from the drop-in-center. That the social contact with other members is on a regular basis is demonstrated first by most respondents saying "hi" to an average of more than 5 other members and talking to more than four other members daily. These numbers are not only substantial; they are also similar to each other. Thus, four out of 5 times a respondent greeted someone else from the community; they stopped and talked to each other. Thus, the majority of the social contact between members does not appear superficial or transient.

The data regarding daily interactions at the drop-in-center reveal that the center is visited on a little more than a third of the total days. However, given that the center is not open on the weekends, it seems more meaningful to point out that it is visited on approximately half of the reported weekdays. Thus, it seems that it is used quite frequently by community members. This frequency of use is quite notable given the physical space which was occupied by the drop-in-center at the time of the data collection. During this time the drop-in-center, including the space set aside for members to congregate and the offices of several staff, was housed in approximately 800 square feet of office space. That such a basic facility was used so frequently by so many underscores the minimum amount of physical space that universities and colleges would be required to provide for their own recovery communities.

What also is remarkable is the amount of time members spent there. Once they dropped in, they stayed—in most cases at least a half hour, but in many cases an hour or two. Based on these numbers, it would appear that members use the drop-in-center as a safe place to be between classes. This information strongly suggest that while they may not need to provide an elaborate physical space for a community to be successful, it seems critical that universities or colleges provide some type of designated and exclusive meeting place. This meeting place provides a safe place where members can always find people, who like themselves, understand addiction and the challenges of staying clean and sober on a college campus. So although being in college means exposure to a social context that almost certainly will challenge the sobriety of anyone in recovery, being at a college with a drop-in-center allows people in recovery to control their exposure to this context.

While talks about recovery are more common at the drop-in-center than elsewhere, occurring on 70% of the times when advice was being provided at the drop-in-center, it does not seem that the setting is a recovery-only zone. In fact, like other settings, the most common activity was just hanging out and talking. Among popular topics were past and future social events. In contrast, on only a small fraction of the time spent at the drop-in-center did past treatment and substance use experiences come up.

What is unique about this setting compared to the others examined with diary data is the presence of CSAR staff members. As made clear by the data presented, they play a very active role in the social interactions there. It may be that through their interactions with community members in the drop-in-center that staff can provide guidance to community members, both as individuals and as a community. Moreover, they can keep being apprised of the health of the community members, again both as individuals and as a community. This opportunity to guide and monitor individuals and the community provides an important informal supplement to the seminar setting, which is used as the primary vehicle for teaching members about addictions and recovery. Staff-to-member interactions at the drop-in-center also provide staff members with a great chance to build rapport with community members.

Good News: Near Constant Contact with Community Members Outside of Center

The most striking information provided by the diary data regards the vast amounts of time members spend with each other outside the drop-in-center. Social time with community members happens on most days and nearly always stretches into several hours. By being there to just to hang out with, to eat lunch with while on campus, to share dinner with while at home, and to watch TV and DVDs with, it seems that other members provide a nearly omnipresent abstinence supportive network. Thus, just as much as the drop-in-center provides members with a safe place while on campus during the day, it seems that other members provide a similarly safe context for each other while off campus.

Reponses also suggest that members provide each other with their closest friends—those with whom they are most likely to have deep conversations. That the environment that these friends provide is protective is suggested by two findings. First, these friends are the most likely to go with them to dry parties. In fact, the extent of the abstinence friendly social network is what provides such dry parties. By creating this context, where respondents can "party" without drinking and drugging, these friends provide a crucial role. And second, they are also likely to accompany respondents when they go to bars and parties where substances are being used.

Of the three groups examined, respondents spent the least amount of days with noncommunity 12-step people. In some ways, social time with these friends was similar to social time with community friends. For example, the percentages of days that included heavy emotional talk (21%) and in which topics were discussed in terms of recovery (50%) was the same for social time spent with community and noncommunity friends. However, in terms of frequency of contact and the duration of contact time with these friends, this friendship group was very different. Respondents only spent time with them on about 1/3 of days and when they spent time with them were not very likely to have lunch or dinner, or to watch TV or DVDs with them. It seems that these friends play a different role in the lives of community members. They are less central to their daily lives. Although they are also in recovery, they do not provide or occupy the primary social contexts in which the respondents spend their days. Their importance should not be minimized, however. They may provide important perspectives on recovery that may not be available inside the collegiate community. They may also provide an opportunity to honestly talk about the community and a respondents place and perspectives about it, without the conversations getting back to other members.

Moreover, social interaction with noncommunity members is most likely the best practice they will have for maintaining similar abstinence-supportive relationships once they graduate. Although the social network of other community members provides the primary support for abstinence within the Collegiate Recovery Community, one reasonable concern is that members can become overly reliant upon it. To the extent that members become dependent on the fellowship of the

CRC it could bode poorly for their ability to sustain recovery after leaving the community. Therefore, the importance of building and maintaining relationships with noncommunity 12-step members is emphasized.

Members of the community also spend time with fellow college students who are not in recovery. Socialization with such individuals occurred on 44% of reported days. Unlike time with community members, which is easy to view as protective—in fact, such time is viewed as the reason why the community exists; it is difficult to know if 45% of days are the "correct" amount of time for members to spend with people who are not in recovery. Of course, it is not the intent of the community to isolate its members from the larger college community. But just like it is important for members to develop their skills in building and maintaining relationships with noncommunity recovery members during their time within the CRC, it is also important that they develop friendships and working relationships with people who are not in recovery. After all, most of their social worlds when they graduate from college will be in settings with nonrecovery people. This is especially true for their work lives, where they will have to interact with and form friendships with people who are not in recovery. If they do not develop the ability to interact with normies while they are surrounded by the protective context of the community, they will be at a high risk for relapse once they graduate.

At first glance, going to bars and parties with substance use may be perplexing. However, just like these students view going to football and basketball games as part of the college experience, they also view going to bars and parties as part of the normative and necessary social life of college. There is something to this view—as after college they will be in many social settings where there will be drinking. It is naïve to think that they will be able to avoid such settings. Thus it is better that they learn how to participate in these activities without succumbing to the temptation to drink or use drugs during their time as members of the recovery community. What may help them participate in these activities but do so as safely as possible is that they are likely to go to these bars and wet parties with other community members. The presence of these members may serve as a buffer, helping to minimize their contact with drinking others when they go out to dance and see bands.

In addition to providing a buffer between individual members and temptations, being with other members no doubt provides support for the decision not to drink when the offer of alcohol does occur. As provided above, being offered alcohol was a common experience. More than half of respondents reported being offered such during the short duration of their data collection flight. And, nearly 20% reported being offered alcohol fairly regularly (on 5 days or more). The frequency of this occurrence underscores how potentially difficult a college experience can be for young adults in recovery. Even surrounded by the protective context of the recovery community, many members are regularly being confronted by opportunities to use substances.

Considering these opportunities to drink, it is a good thing that members are so involved in "working" their 12-step program; by attending 12-step meetings, applying steps to their daily lives, talking to their sponsors (which occurs on nearly half of the total days), and reading 12-step literature. Taken together, these daily behaviors paint a picture of a community of young men and women have embraced the 12-step lifestyle.

Some Bad News

In the midst of what appears to be a lot of very positive news—time at the drop-in-center, time with community members outside the center, additional abstinence support from 12-step affiliates who are not associated with the Collegiate Recovery Center, evidence that members are activity "working" their recovery programs, as well as what seems to be developmentally appropriate associations with nonrecovery friends and participation in college activities—there is bad news. The bad news is the smoking behaviors of the members. Smoking was common across respondents and days. In most cases it also began early in the morning and involved a $\frac{1}{2}$ pack or more a day. This type of tobacco use is very culturally accepted among the 12-step community. Perhaps members are using tobacco to reduce their cravings or otherwise deal with stress. Regardless of its acceptability in the 12-step culture or how it is being used, it is clearly a health risk to participating members.

Conclusions

By applying daily diary methods to capture the experiences of community members this chapter has demonstrated the degree and depth to which CRC membership is interwoven in the lives of its members. In brief, these methods demonstrate membership provides a web of social support for abstinence that provides both near constant contact with the "fellowship" of the community and access to a support system that can be called upon day or night to get through difficult times. This ubiquity is important because it provides constant reinforcement that people support your recovery and a normalization of your experiences. One thing is clear: members of the Collegiate Recovery Community do not have to make it on their own.

References

Almeida, D. M. (2005). Resilience and vulnerability to daily stressors assessed via diary methods. *Current Directions in Psychological Science, 14*(2), 62–68.

Armeli, S., Carney, M. A., Tennen, H., Affleck, G., & O'Neal, T. P. (2000). Stress and alcohol use: A daily process examination of the stressor-vulnerability model. *Journal of Personality and Social Psychology, 78,* 979–994.

Beattie, M. C., & Longabaugh, R. (1997). Interpersonal factors and post-treatment drinking and subjective well-being. *Addiction, 93,* 1507–1521.

Bolger, N., Davis, A., & Rafaeli, E. (2003). Diary methods: Capturing life as it is lived. *Annual Review of Psychology, 54*(579), 616.

Bolger, N., DeLongis, A., Kessler, R. C., & Schilling, E. A. (1989). Effects of daily stress on negative mood. *Journal of Personality and Social Psychology, 57,* 808.

Bond, J., Kaskutas, L. A., & Weisner, C. (2003). The persistent influence of social networks and alcoholics anonymous on abstinence. *Journal of Studies on Alcohol, 64,* 579–588.

Cleveland, H. H., Harris, K. S., Baker, A., Herbert, R., & Dean, L. R. (2007). Characteristics of a collegiate recovery community: Safe haven in an abstinence hostile collegiate environment. *Journal of Substance Abuse Treatment, 33,* 13–23.

Humphreys, K., Mankowski, E. S., Moos, R., & Finney, J. W. (1999). Do enhanced friendship networks and active coping mediate the effects of self-help groups on substance abuse? *Annals of Behavioral Medicine, 21,* 54–60.

Humphreys, K., & Noke, J. M. (1997). The influence of posttreatment mutual help group participation on the friendship networks of substance abuse patients. *American Journal of Community Psychology, 25,* 1–17.

Longabaugh, R., & Beattie, M. C. (1986). Social investment, environmental support, and treatment outcomes of alcoholics. *Alcohol Health Research World, 10,* 64–66.

Longabaugh, R., Wirtz, P. W., Zweben, A., & Stout, R. L. (1998). Network support for drinking, alcoholics Anonymous, and Longterm matching. *Addiction, 93,* 1313–1333.

Mohr, C. D., Armeli, S., Tennen, H., Carney, M. A., Affleck, G., & Hromi, A. (2001). Daily interpersonal experiences, context, and alcohol consumption: Crying in your beer and toasting good times. *Journal of Personality and Social Psychology, 80,* 489–500.

Tonigan, J. S., Ashcroft, F., & Miller, W. R. (1995). AA group dynamics and 12-step activity. *Journal of Studies on Alcohol, 56,* 616–621.

Chapter 7
How Membership in the Collegiate Recovery Community Maximizes Social Support for Abstinence and Reduces Risk of Relapse

H. Harrington Cleveland, Richard P. Wiebe, and Jacquelyn D. Wiersma

According to the National Center on Addiction and Substance Abuse (CASA) at Columbia University, a 2005 survey revealed that 68% of full-time American college students (vs. 59% of nonstudents) reported alcohol use within the past month, with 83% having drunk within the past year. For illicit drugs, 37% of students reported use within the past year (CASA, 2007). In this risky environment, with both substances and users widely available, it is especially important for students who wish to recover from drug and alcohol problems to have a safe place in which to do so. The principal mission of the Center for the Study of Addiction and Recovery (CSAR) at Texas Tech University (TTU) is to provide such an environment for young men and women who wish to maintain abstinence and build a strong recovery while pursuing a college education (CSAR, 2008). To this end, the CSAR runs the College Recovery Community (CRC), described more fully in Chapters 1 and 2 of this volume, which is intended to provide a "recovery-safe" social network.

A major part of a context being safe for continued abstinence is the extent to which it maximizes the number of abstinent safe vs. abstinent risky individuals in the social networks of people in recovery. In evaluating the degree to which membership in the CRC translates into such a safe context, this chapter focuses on three tasks. The first is to review the extant literature about social support and social networks as they influence recovery, in order to identify important goals for the social support component of a recovery program for young adults in recovery in a college context. The second is to present data and analyses that examine the relative levels of support for abstinence and risk for relapse that exist within the social networks of CRC members. And the third is to examine these findings in light of the goals identified in the literature review. As shall be seen, although the CRC has not completely eliminated substance-using friends from the social networks of its members, it does appear to have succeeded in providing a relatively safe environment for recovery.

H.H. Cleveland (✉)
The Pennsylvania State University, University Park, PA, USA
e-mail: cleveland@psu.edu

H.H. Cleveland et al. (eds.), *Substance Abuse Recovery in College*, Advancing
Responsible Adolescent Development, DOI 10.1007/978-1-4419-1767-6_7,
© Springer Science+Business Media, LLC 2010

Social Networks and Social Support

Social networks and social support are linked concepts. Social networks are the organizations or relationships that constitute the social context around individuals, such as friends and family. It is through these networks that people can receive the appraisals of value and the assistance that collectively constitutes social support. Perhaps as a result, individuals with supportive social networks have generally higher physical and psychological health and well-being than those who do not (Cohen & Willis, 1985). Social support appears especially important for people in recovery from substance use addictions. Without it, their likelihood of maintaining abstinence is substantially reduced (Beattie et al., 1993).

For people in recovery, not all social support is created equal. The most important distinction is between *general* social support and *abstinence-specific* (also known as substance-specific or alcohol-specific) social support (Beattie & Longabaugh, 1999; Wasserman, Stewart, & Delucchi, 2001). Further, both general and abstinence-specific support may be examined in at least two different ways: structural and functional (Beattie & Longabaugh, 1997; Wasserman et al., 2001). This scheme results in four types of support: general structural, abstinence-specific structural, general functional, and abstinence-specific functional.

To measure general structural support, researchers have examined the quantity of supportive significant others—friends, family—in the individual's social network. To measure abstinence-specific structural support, they have examined the ratio of abstinent to substance-using significant others. In contrast, functional support involves the perceived or actual assistance offered by significant others (the quality of support may also be measured; Beattie and Longabaugh (1997)). Clearly, these concepts overlap: All things being equal, the greater the number of abstinent individuals in your network, the greater potential for actual support. However, it is also possible that a great deal of actual assistance can be offered by relatively few individuals or, conversely, that an individual in recovery may be isolated from significant others who could provide, but are not currently providing, assistance.

General functional support is the assistance that people receive to help them negotiate overall life goals. Research on alcoholics has found that this type of support enhances self-confidence and self-esteem, and has a direct impact on health and well-being (Beattie & Longabaugh, 1999). Addicts can receive general support from any member of their social network, regardless of their substance use status (Procidano & Heller, 1983). However, although it may enhance self-esteem, a general support structure that includes substance-using significant others can endanger recovery (Goehl, Nunes, Quitkin, & Hilton, 1993; Riehman, Wechsberg, Zule, Lam, & Levine, 2008).

In contrast, abstinence-specific functional support directly addresses the addiction itself and can include strategies to maintain abstinence. Because of its nature, it is usually received from friends and family who are abstinent themselves (Beattie & Longabaugh, 1999; Wasserman et al., 2001). As the goal of the CRC is to facilitate abstinence and not merely self-esteem, the CRC concentrates on enhancing members' abstinence-specific support networks.

This chapter considers the characteristics of the CRC members' social support networks in terms of the abstinence-specific support they provide compared with the relapse risk they present. Members of the CRC differ in several ways from participants in most alcohol research. Not only are they younger and have longer recoveries than participants in most studies in this research area, but their addictions are to both alcohol and other drugs (see   Chapter 4). Thus, it is appropriate to speak of abstinence-specific, rather than simply alcohol-specific, support.

Although most studies about social support and recovery use samples of middle-aged adults who are beginning their recovery from alcoholism, studies of people addicted to cocaine (Galanter, Dermatis, Keller, & Trujillo, 2002), crack cocaine (Riehman et al., 2008), opioids (Goehl et al., 1993; van den Brink & Haansen, 2006), and a mix of substances, either alone (Davis & Jason, 2005) or in conjunction with another mental health problem (Laudet, Cleland, Magura, Vogel, & Knight, 2004), are mainly consonant with the alcohol literature. The same conclusion seems to apply regardless of the substance used: If abstinence is the goal, then the network should contain abstainers who actively support recovery and should not contain active users or alcohol or other drugs. In this chapter, we will refer to all network support targeted specifically toward helping the addict maintain recovery, regardless of substance, as abstinence-specific, but will identify studies that deal specifically with alcohol as well as highlight any conflicts among studies that examine addiction to different substances.

The alcoholism literature has established that although both general and abstinence-specific support can be beneficial, abstinence-specific support seems to be more effective in facilitating long-term abstinence. General social support appears most important in the short-term and can enhance the effectiveness of abstinence-specific support (Beattie & Longabaugh, 1997). But general support can be a two-edged sword. As it often comes from friends and family who are drinkers themselves, general support can be sometimes be associated with relapse risk (Gordon & Zrull, 1991). In fact, one of the best predictors of relapse is the number of drinkers in an alcoholic's social network of regular contacts a year following treatment (Bond, Kaskutas, & Weisner, 2003). Perhaps this is why alcoholics tend to have better outcomes with the presence of strong and supportive abstinent significant others (Beattie et al., 1993; Longabaugh & Beattie, 1985). Similar results have been found for methadone addicts; those with at least one drug user in their social networks were 63% likely to test positive for use, vs. only 35% for those with no close users in their networks (Goehl et al., 1993).

Alcohol's ubiquity, both in general society and on college campuses, renders it unlikely that an individual can completely excise drinkers from his or her social network; this can also be true in some contexts for other drugs (Riehman et al., 2008). To deal with this phenomenon, abstinence-specific support can provide specific strategies—for example, feedback from other alcoholics—for maintaining abstinence in the face of a drinking society. The most notable source of abstinence-specific support for alcoholics is through their affiliation with Alcoholics Anonymous (AA). Alcoholics Anonymous serves as a reference and support group to buffer a person from the negative effects of social members' networks who may drink themselves. Such "safe" social network members can provide not only specific information about techniques to avoid relapse, but also evidence that sustained recovery is possible. Thus, AA provides both structural and functional abstinence-specific support.

It is clear that both structural and functional abstinence-specific supports are associated with enhanced likelihood of continued abstinence. Alcoholics with more abstainers or recovering alcoholics in their support networks have better outcomes (Zywiak, Longabaugh, & Wirtz, 2002). In addition, the more contact they have with abstinent network members and the more importance they place on them, the greater likelihood they will use these supportive influences. These abstinent friends appear to facilitate recovery both because they provide abstinent-supportive replacements for old substance-using friends (Humphreys & Noke, 1997) and because they mitigate the influence of remaining substance using friends (Bond et al., 2003).

Both having abstinent friends and having abstinent friends who participate in AA appear to help maintain recovery. Kaskutas, Bond, and Humphrey (2002) found that 78% of those with AA abstinent friends in their support group were able to stay sober at least 30 days and 72% stayed sober for at least 90 days. Approximately 52% of alcoholics who had non-AA abstinent friends were able to stay sober at least 30 days, with 45% staying sober for 90 days. However, only 37% of alcoholics whose social network provided *no* abstinent friends stayed sober for 30 days and only 33% stayed sober for 90 days. Presumably, the friends in AA are helping to deliver abstinence-related interventions, thus providing functional as well as structural support.

The importance of social support may depend on the length of recovery, as individuals early in their recovery may have a harder time with staying sober without social network support for abstinence. In one study of polydrug users in a community home-based recovery program, length of stay in the program was positively related to "abstinence self-efficacy," an internal resource facilitating abstinence (Davis & Jason, 2005). See Chapter 5 for more information on self-efficacy and CRC members. Thus, the social support needed for people with relatively established recoveries, such as longer term members of the CRC, may differ from those who are just beginning the recovery process. Relatively newly recovered addicts, even if members of the CRC, may have a greater need for abstinence-specific support in their networks.

In summary, research has demonstrated that characteristics of social networks of those successfully maintaining abstinence include the following: (a) a higher proportion of nondrinking members (Mohr, Averna, Kenny, & Del Boca, 2001); (b) more contact with a nondrinking member (Booth et al., 1992); (c) more investment in relationships with nondrinking members (Zywiak et al., 2002), and (d) ranking more nondrinkers as "most important" (Mohr et al., 2001). The greater availability, proximity, and importance of nondrinking network members increases the potential for functional support and successful recovery.

Sex Differences

Males and females in recovery may both have different social network risks and be differently challenged by these risks. Specifically, differences in networks appear to place males more at risk. Among recovering alcoholics, being male, young, and early in recovery were all related to having drinking friends and spending more time with them (Mohr et al., 2001). Because men are more likely to hang out with other men, and men are generally more likely than women to drink, their social networks are more likely to place them at risk for relapsing. In contrast, females generally have less risky social networks. Moreover, even when females begin treatment with drinking friends whom they rate among their most important friends, they are more likely to drop these friends from the list of most important friends as they stay in recovery. Thus, females appear more willing than males to change their social networks to safeguard their recovery.

Two recent studies cloud the picture. In their study of polydrug users, Davis and Jason (2005) found that social support variables completely mediated the relationship between length of program stay and abstinence self-efficacy among females, but not males, suggesting that internal supports for abstinence are more closely tied to social support among women than men. And in a study of out-of-treatment crack users, Riehman and colleagues (2008) found social support variables to be unrelated to crack use among females, but that males with abstinent partners were themselves less likely to use.

Support and the CRC

In general, the research reveals that abstinence-specific social support, both structural and functional, strongly predicts successful recovery. Providing such support is one of the primary reasons the CSAR has established the CRC at TTU. Because most CRC members are traditionally aged college students, and college is a context with a social environment organized around drinking, they may have an increased risk of having social networks that contain drinking friends. As friends appear to have greater impact than family on recovering alcoholics (Beattie & Longabaugh, 1997; Rosenberg, 1983), being nested inside this potential drinking context may be particularly dangerous for those young adults. Thus, the composition of CRC members' immediate social networks seems critically important for their sustained recoveries. This raises the question: Although the CRC provides its members with potentially "safe" (i.e., abstaining) people, do they incorporate these safe members into their social networks or do they populate their networks with potentially risky (i.e., drinking) members? And, even if they have abstainers in their networks, do they receive functional support from them?

To help answer these questions, we examined the extent to which CRC members' social networks presented both abstinence support and relapse risk. Specifically, we discerned (a) the relative levels of abstainers vs. drinkers/substance users in the CRC

members' social networks (structural abstinence-specific support); (b) the amount
of contact members had with abstainers vs. drinkers; and (c) the abstinent support
vs. relapse risk that is present among the "most important" people within CRC members' social networks. We also examined whether the sex differences that have been
reported in the literature exist within this community.

Method

Respondents

Participants were members of the CRC at TTU from whom data were collected
between March 2004 and November 2004. The initial March 2004 data collection
consisted of 52 respondents. Additional data were collected during the fall of 2004
from another 30 students who had recently joined the CRC that fall. Data from nine
participants who reported their primary addiction as an eating disorder and seven
participants with missing data on the social network measure were excluded from
the analyses reported here, leaving 66 in the final sample. Prior to data collections,
for which IRB approval was obtained, researchers explained to potential participants
that participation was voluntary and that all data were anonymous. All respondents
were full-time college students, with an average age of 23.2 years old, with a range
of 18–53. Nearly all (94%) were Caucasian.

Measures

In the past decade, the primary instrument used to collect data on the social networks
of those in recovery has been from the Inventory of Important People and Activities
(IPA). This instrument was used by Project MATCH (Project MATCH Research
Group, 1997a; 1997b; 1998), a multisite national study that examined the efficacy
of matching treatment methods to client characteristics. The IPA was designed to be
administered to actively using clients in alcohol treatment facilities. As such, the IPA
asked respondents how important social network members reacted to respondents
drinking and how they reacted to respondents not drinking. In contrast, this project
needed the inventory to assess the social networks of people who are in recovery
(i.e., they are not actively using substances) from the abuse of various substances,
not just alcohol. We modified the IPA to assess the social network challenges faced
by people trying to maintain recovery from alcohol and other substances, rather
than those of people who are attempting to stop their active use of alcohol (see also
Davis & Jason, 2005).

Similar to the original IPA, the modified instrument, which we refer to as the
IPA-R (Inventory of Important People and Activities for Recovery), contains three
tables. The first two tables describe the respondents' social networks and the third

table describes respondents' activities. The criteria for inclusion in the social network tables were that individuals listed had to be at least 12 years of age. For the spring 2004 data collection, respondents were asked to use a 6 month timeframe for their social network; however, for the fall 2005 data collections a 3 month timeframe was used to accommodate new members' more recent transition to the CRC. A subset of the items from Tables 7.1 and 7.2 were used to construct variables for this study's analyses, which includes two outcome variables: abstinence support and recovery risk. The maximum number of individuals allowed on the first table was 12. For each individual listed, respondents were asked to specify (a) the relationship of the network member to the respondent, (b) the sex of the network member, (c) the number of years and months known to the network member, (d) frequency of contact, (e) the drinking status of the network member, (f) drinking frequency of the network member, and (g) maximum number of daily drinks for this network member. It should be noted that rather than ask about the drug use behaviors of social network members, we focused on their drinking status. This decision was made based on the belief that the primary relapse risk associated with the college social context is the ubiquity of alcohol use and that the recovery program of members requires them to be abstinent from alcohol.

The second table of the IPA-R asked respondents to identify the four most important members of their social networks. The table asked respondents to list: (a) the identity number for the network member from Table 7.1, (b) the rank from 1 to 4 of the network member in terms of general importance among the four listed, (c) the rank from 1 to 4 of the network member in terms of importance as related to recovery among the four listed, (d) how much the respondent liked the network member (on a scale from 1 "totally disliked" to 7 "totally liked"), (e) how important this network member been to the respondent (on a scale from 1 "not at all" to 6 "extremely important"), (f) how would this network member react to your drinking, (g) how has this person reacted to your not using, (h) how often this person has had a drink around the respondent, (i) how often respondent has talked to this person about respondent's past substance use or current recovery, and (j) if the person was also in recovery, how often has respondent talked to this person about the network members own past substance use or recovery. From these tables, we constructed four measures to assess abstinence-specific support, (a) Total Abstainers, (b) Abstainer Contact, (c) Important Abstainers, and (d) Important Abstainer Contact, and four measures of *Relapse Risk* (a) Total Drinkers, (b) Drinker Contact, (c) Important Drinkers, and (d) Important Drinker Contact.

Total abstainers. This structural measure was derived from Table 7.1, column 6, of the IPA-R. This column asked participants to indicate the drinking/substance use status of network members listed, which included the following: (1) long-term recovering alcoholic or substance user (5 + years); (2) recovering alcoholic/user; (3) abstainer; (4) light drinker; (5) moderate drinker; (6) heavy drinker; and/or (99) don't know. To create the Total Abstainers support measure, the total number of social network members who were long-term recovering, recovering, or abstainers were summed to create an index that could take on a value of zero (indicating no abstainers in the network) to 12.

Table 7.1 Outcome variables for entire sample

Measure	N	Mean	SD	Possible min	Possible max	Sample min	Sample max	Q1	Q3
Abstinence support									
Total abstainers	66	5.86	2.89	0	12	0	12	4	9
Abstainer contact	65	34.18	17.31	0	84	5	84	21	45
Important abstainers	64	2.59	1.22	0	4	0	4	2	4
Important abstainer contact	64	15.89	7.69	0	28	0	28	11	22
Recovery risk									
Total drinkers	66	2.94	2.39	0	12	0	11	1	4
Drinker contact	65	15.95	12.79	0	84	0	52	6	22
Important drinkers	64	1.28	1.16	0	4	0	4	0	2
Important drinker contact	64	7.63	7.34	0	28	0	28	0	12
Size of social network	65	9.12	2.79	0	12	2	12	7	12

Note: $N = 65$.

Table 7.2 Means (*SDs*) of outcome variables by biological sex

	Abstinence support				
	Total abstainers	Abstainer contact	Important abstainers	Important abstainer contact	Size of network
Females (*n* = 23)	5.74 (2.66)	33.13 (19.97)	2.26 (1.10)	14.17 (6.76)	9.35 (2.74)
Males (*n* = 43)	5.93 (2.88)	34.76 (15.89)	2.78 (1.26)	16.85 (8.08)	9.00 (2.84)
	Recovery risk				
	Total drinkers	Drinker contact	Important drinkers	Important drinker contact	Size of network
Females (*n* = 23)	3.35 (2.53)	18.43 (13.59)	1.52 (1.04)	9.39 (7.05)	9.35 (2.74)
Males (*n* = 43)	2.72 (2.30)	14.60 (12.27)	1.15 (1.22)	6.63 (7.40)	9.00 (2.84)

Note: *N* = 66, standard deviations are in parentheses

Abstainer contact. This measure of functional abstinence-specific support was constructed by examining the frequency of contact with all abstainers, as defined above, within the network of each study participant. Column 5 of Table 7.1 of the IPA-R asks participants to indicate the frequency of contact they had with each network member listed, scored as follows: (0) none in past 6 months, (1) once in past 6 months, (2) less than once per month, (3) once per month, (4) every other week, (5) 1–2 days per week, (6) 3–6 days per week, or (7) daily. To create the Abstainer Contact score for each participant, only contacts with abstainers were counted. Each abstainer in the network got a score from 0 (no contact) to 7 (daily), and these scores were summed. The possible range of Abstainer Contact was 0, which would indicate no contact with any abstainers in the past 6 months, to 84, which would indicate a social network of 12 abstainers with whom they had daily contact.

Important abstainers. The third measure of abstinence support was the number of network members listed as "most important" (up to four out of 12) who were also identified as abstainers. This measure combined information from Table 7.1 describing the abstinence status of network members with information from Table 7.2 about which members were among respondents' most important social network. This measure has a possible range of 0 (no abstainers listed as important) to 4 (all four "most important" network members were abstainers, including those in recovery).

Important abstainer contact. An index of contact with important abstainers was created by summing the frequency of contact for all the abstainers in the "most important" social network. Contact frequency for these social network members was summed to produce an Important Abstainer Contact measure, with a range of 0–28. A score of 0 would indicate no contact with any important abstainers, while a score of 28 would indicate daily contact with four important abstainers.

Total drinkers. This measure was used information from column 6 of Table 7.1, which asked respondents to indicate the drinking status of network members listed. To create the Total Drinkers measure, responses that indicated light, moderate, or heavy drinking were summed. The resulting possible range was from 0 to 12, with 0 indicating no drinkers in network and 12 indicating all possible network members were drinkers.

Drinker contact. The second measure of relapse risk was the sum of contact frequency for all the drinkers in the social network. Contact frequency for each drinker in the social network was summed to create a Drinker Contact index, with a possible range of 0 (indicating no contact with any drinkers in the past 6 months) to 84 (indicating a social network of 12 drinkers with whom respondents had daily contact).

Important drinkers. The third social network relapse risk measure tallied the number of drinkers within the individuals whom respondents listed as "most important" to them, up to a maximum of 4.

Important drinker contact. The fourth measure is the sum of contact frequency with important drinkers. Like the Important Abstainer Contact measure, the potential range of this measure was 0–28, with 0 indicating no contact with any important drinkers in the past 6 months and 28 indicating daily contact with 4 important drinkers.

Results

Table 7.1 provides the grand means, standard deviations, and other descriptive information for the measures of abstinence-specific social support and relapse risk associated with participants' social networks. Due to the correspondence between the construction of the four abstinence-specific support and the four recovery risk measures, pairs of these measures (e.g., Important Abstainers vs. Important Drinkers) have the same possible minimums and maximums. Thus, comparing values across these pairs provides an opportunity to consider the degree of relative support and risk to which members of the Collegiate Recovery Community (CRC) are exposed.

For each pair of indicators, respondents reported greater abstinence support than relapse risk. In fact, within each pair of indicators the means for abstinence support were nearly or more than double of those for the corresponding relapse risk indicator. Specifically the means were as follows: (a) 5.86 for Total Abstainers vs. 2.94 for Total Drinkers, (b) 34.18 for Abstainer Contact vs. 15.95 for User Contact, (c) 2.59 for Important Abstainers vs. 1.28 for Important Drinkers, and (d) 15.89 for Important Abstainer Contact vs. 7.63 for Important User Contact.

The extent of these differences is underscored by the interquartile ranges for these eight measures, which are provided on the far right side of Table 7.1. For the Total Abstainers measure, the lower interquartile (i.e., the 25th percentile) was 4.0, which is the same value as the *upper* quartile range (75th percentile) for Total Drinkers. That the same value defines the 25th percentile of social network protectiveness that defines the 75th percentile of social network risk demonstrates the degree to which CRC members' social networks are populated by protective rather than risky individuals. This same pattern is demonstrated by each of the other three pairs of protective vs. risky network measures. For each of these pairs, the 25th percentile of the abstinence measure has a value similar to the 75th percentile of the mirror image relapse risk indicator. Additional evidence of the degree of differences in abstinence support vs. relapse risk can be gathered by looking at the differences between the measures relative to the standard deviations. In each case, the average mean for relapse risk is more than one standard deviation lower than the corresponding measure of abstinence support.

Another illustration of the protectiveness of the social networks within the CRC is the percentage of the participants' social networks that consisted of abstainers, found by dividing the mean number of abstainers in each network (5.86) by the mean total network size (9.12). This calculation reveals that 65% of CRC members' social networks consisted of "safe" people.

Sex Differences

Sex differences were tested for the four abstinence support outcomes and the four relapse risk outcomes. The raw means and standard deviations by sex are presented in Table 7.2. In contrast to published findings (e.g., Mohr et al., 2001), males, instead of females, reported more abstinent support and less risk. Specifically, males reported higher levels of each of the four abstinence support measures and lower levels of each of the relapse risk measures. However, ANOVAs revealed that these differences, although systematic, were not significant.

Discussion

The research is clear: Stocking one's social network with abstainers is an important correlate of successful recovery (Beattie & Longabaugh, 1997, 1999). And this is particularly difficult to do in an American university, where 68% of students are likely to have used alcohol within the past month, and 37% to have used illicit drugs within the past year (CASA, 2007). The data and analyses reported in this chapter provide strong evidence that the CRC does in fact provide a protective milieu for young adults in recovery from alcohol and other substance use problems, by, among other things, giving them the opportunity to construct safe social networks.

Importantly, CRC members appear to have taken advantage of this opportunity. Their social networks are dominated by abstinent individuals, containing nearly twice as many abstainers as drinkers, with whom they have more than twice as much contact than with drinkers. Their lists of important individuals within these networks are also dominated by abstainers with twice as many abstainers in the network and twice as much contact with abstainers. This is strikingly different from the overall proportion of drinkers and substance users in American colleges and universities, where more than twice as many students use than abstain (CASA, 2007). With 65% of their social networks consisting of "safe" members, CRC members enjoy a protective social context that would be encouraging anywhere. That the CRC can provide such a safe environment for young adults in recovery who are attending a large university is dramatic evidence of the CSAR's success in providing safeguards to protect these young adults' recoveries.

The degree to which the CRC helps protect its members from the otherwise abstinence-hostile social context of college is also evident in the lack of differences found between male and female members' social network abstinence support and relapse risk. Most studies have found that males' social network relapse risk is consistently higher (Mohr et al., 2001). However, it appears that the CRC's environment is so protective that it essentially creates a protective ceiling effect, blocking males' tendency to construct social networks filled with drinking friends and creating a statistical equivalence between males and females. In fact, males reported more abstinent friends and more contact with them, and fewer drinking friends and contact with them than did females, although the difference is not statistically significant.

This gender difference may be due, in part, to the positive ratio of males to females in the community. It appears that by providing males so many abstinent same-sex peers with whom to form friendships, the CRC may be able to counteract males' tendency to construct riskier social networks by making the raw materials for safe networks—other abstaining males—readily available (Beattie & Longabaugh, 1999).

Thus, along with its programming, discussed in detail elsewhere (see Chapters 2, 3, and 9) and the mere fact of its existence, the comparatively large size of the CRC may be very important in facilitating recovery. At the time of data collection, the CRC had over 50 members. With so many age-matched abstinent peers readily available, it seems that CRC members have an unusual opportunity to stock their social networks with abstainers compared with individuals in smaller recovery communities or at institutions with no recovery community whatsoever.

Success through numbers is consistent with social identity theory (Barber, Eccles, & Stone, 2001), discussed in Chapter 3 . The CRC provides young college students, of both sexes, recovering from addictions the opportunity to identify with a substantial number of people like themselves within the context of a salient, attractive, and stable group. This social identity may be reinforced by cultural symbols and rituals associated with recovery within the ecological context of the CRC, strengthening the tendency of both male and female members to identify with and commit to the group (Matto, 2004). As Chapter 3 notes, fellow group members are generally high academic achievers, enhancing the sense that the group and its members are special—they're not simply surviving, they're thriving.

Overall, the fact that CRC members' networks include so many abstinent people appears important because it increases the availability of functional social support from individuals who understand the process of recovery (Groh, Jason, & Keys, 2008), which can help them deal with its day-to-day challenges, as discussed in Chapter 6, and construct a mature, prosocial, and sober identity, as discussed in Chapter 3. As collegiate recovery communities become more common in colleges and universities across the country, it will be possible to examine whether such communities are subject to a size threshold: a minimum number of members needed to provide them with enough safe people for their social networks.

Conclusions

In recognition that social support is the key ingredient to sustained abstinence, the CSAR designed the CRC so that its members can have access to others in recovery while attending college. Prior to the analyses presented here, however, it was not clear just how effectively membership in the CRC both provides support for abstinence and protect against relapse risk by reducing the numbers of drinking individuals within members social networks. In short, CRC membership populates members' social networks with "safe" individuals while simultaneously reducing the number of "risky" members. Specifically, across four different measures of social network abstinence support and relapse risk, CRC members enjoy twice or nearly twice the numbers of and contact with safe vs. risky social network members.

When considering different models of collegiate recovery support, it is hard to imagine that programs with substantially smaller communities would be as effective in delivering this level of support.

References

Barber, B., Eccles, J., & Stone, M. (2001). Whatever happened to the Jock, the Brain, and the Princess? Young adult pathways linked to adolescent activity involvement and social identity (2001). *Journal of Adolescent Research, 16*(5), 429–455.

Beattie, M., & Longabaugh, R. (1997). Interpersonal factors and post-treatment drinking and subjective wellbeing. *Addiction, 92*, 1507–1521.

Beattie, M., & Longabaugh, R. (1999). General and alcohol-specific social support following treatment. *Addictive Behaviors, 24*, 593–606.

Beattie, M., Longabaugh, R., Elliot, G., Stout, R., Fava, J., & Noel, N. (1993). Effect of the social environment on alcohol involvement and subjective well-being prior to alcoholism treatment. *Journal of Studies on Alcohol, 54*, 283–296.

Bond, J., Kaskutas, L. A., & Weisner, C. (2003). The persistent influence of social networks and Alcoholics Anonymous on abstinence. *Journal of Studies on Alcohol, 64*, 579–588.

Booth, B. M., Russell, D. W., Soucek, S., & Laughlin, P. R. (1992). Social support and outcome of alcohol treatment: An exploratory analysis. *American Journal of Drug and Alcohol Abuse, 18*(1), 87–102.

Center for the Study of Addiction and Recovery (CSAR) (2008). *Goals and purpose of the Center.* Retrieved on February 24, 2008, from http://www.depts.ttu.edu/hs/csa/Goals%20Page.html.

Cohen, S., & Willis, T. A. (1985). Stress, social support, and the buffering hypothesis. *Psychology Bulletin, 98*, 310–357.

Davis, M. I., & Jason, L. A. (2005). Sex differences in social support and self-efficacy within a recovery community. *American Journal of Community Psychology, 36*, 259–274.

Galanter, M., Dermatis, H., Keller, D., & Trujillo, M. (2002). Network therapy for cocaine abuse: Use of family and peer supports. *American Journal on Addictions, 11*, 161–166.

Goehl, L., Nunes, E., Quitkin, F., & Hilton, I. (1993). Social networks and methadone treatment outcomes: The costs and benefits of social ties. *American Journal of Drug & Alcohol Abuse, 19*, 252–262.

Gordon, A., & Zrull, M. (1991). Social networks and recovery: One year after inpatient treatment. *Journal of Substance Abuse Treatment, 8*, 143–152.

Groh, D. R., Jason, L. A., & Keys, C. B. (2008). Social network variables in Alcoholics Anonymous: A literature review. *Clinical Psychology Review, 28*, 430–450.

Humphreys, K., & Noke, J. M. (1997). The influence of posttreatment mutual help group participation on the friendship networks of substance abuse patients. *American Journal of Community Psychology, 25*, 1–17.

Kaskutas, L., Bond, J., & Humphreys, K. (2002). Social networks as mediators of the effect of Alcoholics Anonymous. *Addiction, 97*, 891–900.

Laudet, A. B., Cleland, C. M., Magura, S., Vogel, H. S., & Knight, E. L. (2004). Social support mediates the effects of dual-focus mutual aid groups on abstinence from substance use. *American Journal of Community Psychology, 34*, 175–185.

Longabaugh, R., & Beattie, M. C. (1985). *Maximizing the cost-effectiveness of treatment for alcohol abusers.* NIAAA Research Monograph-15, DHHS Publication No. 85-1322. Washington, DC: US Government Printing Office.

Matto, H. (2004). Applying an ecological framework to understanding drug addiction and recovery. *Journal of Social Work Practice in the Addictions, 4*, 5–22.

Mohr, C., Averna, S., Kenny, D., & Del Boca, F. (2001). "Getting by (or getting high) with a little help from my friends": An examination of adult alcoholics' friendships. *Journal of Studies on Alcohol, 62*, 637–645.

National Center on Addiction and Substance Abuse (CASA) (2007). *Wasting the best and brightest: Substance abuse at America's colleges and universities*. New York: Columbia University.

Procidano, M. E., & Heller, K. (1983). Measures of perceived social support from friends and from family. *American Journal of Community Psychology, 11*, 1–24.

Project MATCH Research Group (1997a). Matching alcoholism treatments to client heterogeneity: Project MATCH posttreatment drinking outcomes. *Journal of Studies on Alcohol, 58*, 7–29.

Project MATCH Research Group (1997b). Matching alcoholism treatment to client heterogeneity: Tests of the Project MATCH secondary *a priori* hypotheses. *Addiction, 92*, 1671–1698.

Project MATCH Research Group (1998). Matching alcoholism treatments to client heterogeneity: Treatment main effects and matching effects on drinking during treatment. *Journal of Studies on Alcohol, 59*(6), 631–639.

Riehman, K. S., Wechsberg, W. M., Zule, W., Lam, W. K. K., & Levine, B. (2008). Gender differences in the impact of social support on crack use among African Americans. *Substance Use & Misuse, 43*, 85–104.

Rosenberg, H. (1983). Relapsed vs. non-relapsed alcohol abusers: Coping skills, life events, and social support. *Addictive Behaviors, 8*, 183–186.

van den Brink, W., & Haasen, C. (2006). Evidence-based treatment of opioid-dependent patients. *Canadian Journal of Psychiatry, 51*, 635–646. Weisner et al., 2002.

Wasserman, D. A., Stewart, A. L., & Delucchi, K. L. (2001). Social support and abstinence from opiates and cocaine during opioid maintenance treatment. *Drug and Alcohol Dependence, 65*, 65–75.

Zywiak, W., Longabaugh, R., & Wirtz, P. (2002). Decomposing the relationships between pretreatment social network characteristics and alcohol treatment outcome. *Journal of Studies on Alcohol, 63*, 114–121.

Chapter 8
Building Support for Recovery into an Academic Curriculum: Student Reflections on the Value of Staff Run Seminars

Ann M. Casiraghi and Miriam Mulsow

Collegiate recovery programs, such as the one administered by the Center for the Study of Addiction and Recovery (CSAR) at Texas Tech University (TTU), are expected to provide recovering students with support for both recovery and academic success. In addition to the support provided by a community of fellow recovering students, community members receive resources from specific program services that are delivered primarily by CSAR administration and staff. This chapter presents a program evaluation of one of the major program components of the CSAR program: The Seminar for Recovering Students (Seminar). The goal of this evaluation was to provide information about how students were experiencing Seminar and the value they perceived they were drawing from it. As the Collegiate Recovery Community had grown dramatically, from approximately 25 to over 80 students, under the direction of Dr. Kitty Harris, the CSAR administration believed it was particularly important to determine whether existing program components, such as Seminar, which were designed at time before the expansion of the CRC, were meeting the needs of current community members. This chapter reviews the findings from this evaluation and provides a measure of social support for recovery in the collegiate context piloted during this project modifiable for use in similar recovery maintenance programs. Prior to setting out specific findings, we review the short- and long-term goals of the CSAR program, set out the types of social support that the program is designed to provide, how different program components address these types of social support, and explain the role of Seminar in addressing these social support needs.

Program Goals and Theory

According to CSAR staff, the CRC has three primary program goals: (a) to lay a foundation for long-term and sustained recovery, (b) to provide a context wherein

A.M. Casiraghi (✉)
Texas Tech University, Lubbock, TX, USA
e-mail: anne.m.casiraghi@ttu.edu

H.H. Cleveland et al. (eds.), *Substance Abuse Recovery in College*, Advancing
Responsible Adolescent Development, DOI 10.1007/978-1-4419-1767-6_8,
© Springer Science+Business Media, LLC 2010

community members can safely pursue their educations, and (c) to instill character within students to help them function in society. The CSAR hopes to accomplish these goals by helping CRC members construct prosocial and pro-recovery individual identities (see Chapter 3) and establish social identities as members of a functioning college-based recovery community. For the reasons discussed in Chapter 2 by Harris et al., this volume, these tasks require more than merely providing recovering college students access to 12-step programs. At the core of the CSAR's program theory is the belief that college students in recovery benefit from a social support system that is designed specifically for recovering college students.

The CSAR assumes that as CRC members achieve program goals of staying in recovery and attaining a quality education they develop in other areas. Along with offering opportunities for students to obtain educational support from university service providers, CSAR staff, and fellow CSAR participants, CRC members are encouraged to improve their physical health by staying clean and sober and by practicing general self-care. Additionally, through the character-building process that CSAR is designed to provide, students are expected to learn life skills that allow them to cope with everyday stress without using substances. Finally, the CSAR supports CRC members' development of personal identities, with the hope that when students graduate from the community they will have established a strong sense of life purpose. Although the CSAR is intended to provide all community members with support in each of these areas, staff members realize that there are limits to what they can provide students and that much of the enthusiasm to engage in the program is based on members' own motivation.

An assumption that underlies the CSAR program theory is that successfully completing the program leads to not only continued success in recovery from substances, but also well-being in other areas of life such as intimate relationships, employment, and positive engagement in society. The CSAR staff holds the belief that sustained recovery and a college education potentially paves the way for success with family relationships, possibly deterring the cycle of addiction that tends to run in families. The background developmental theory of young adult recovery, as described in Chapter 3, appears to fit well within the CSAR's overall program theory identified by the evaluation. Both this young adult development and recovery theory, as described in Chapter 2, and the social support focus of the CSAR program emphasize the importance of young adults' social contexts. The young adult development and recovery theory recognizes the significance of the social contexts associated with both adolescent peer relationships during prior addictive behaviors and young adult relationships in recovery. The CSAR program emphasizes the importance of staff in building and supporting a community that supports both recovery from substance abuse and socioemotional development.

Short-term goals. The CSAR staff hold the view that recovery maintenance is the primary short-term program goal. Just as recovery has social aspects, so does relapse. Along with the negative effects on the individual, relapse can negatively affect other CRC members. If a community member relapses, other members might experience emotional distress, increasing their risk of relapse. The CRC facilitates the development of close friendships between recovering students, and students often rely on other members for companionship in recreational and leisure activities. Even though the CRC strives to provide an abstinence-supportive environment for recovering students, inevitably, a small percentage of CSAR students relapse. Accordingly, CSAR staff members vigilantly focus on individual students' commitment to the recovery process.

Relapse can also have adverse effects on academic performance, the second short-term program goal. When recovery is maintained, most CSAR participants succeed academically, as described in Chapter 4. In general, CSAR participants tend to have higher grade point averages than Texas Tech students who are not affiliated with the CSAR. Some CSAR students may have a more difficult time achieving high grade point averages but they tend to possess the commitment and the resiliency to overcome obstacles by adopting a "whatever it takes" mindset.

Relapse can also interfere with the third short-term goal, students' development and use of life skills necessary to maintain their recovery and building healthy and supportive relationships with family members and with friends. Prior to sobriety and entering the CSAR program many members years of addictions and struggles maintaining abstinence had undermined not only their self-confidence and self-esteem, but also their personal relationships, especially those outside the recovery community. The goal of developing and using life skills to forge and maintain personal relationships assumes that the life skills learned and practiced during participation in the CRC will allow members to build and support personal relationships when they leave the CRC community.

Long-term goals. The long-term goals of the CSAR are for graduating students to have lasting continued recovery, maintenance of physical and mental health, and a foundation for building healthy relationships. In essence, the long-term goals are a continuation of the short-term goals but they occur at a deeper level, reflecting the maturity that comes with long-term recovery and development of the self. Accomplishing these goals should improve the chances for CSAR graduates to attain personal and professional achievement, making them more apt to be productive members of society. Ideally, graduates of the program would continue to serve their communities by contributing to society in some capacity. These contributions can take the form of employment, volunteerism, or financial donations.

Social Support

One of the primary tools used by the CSAR to assist community members in their recovery, as well as their overall academic and personal development, is social support. Social support, particularly support directly related to abstinence (Beattie & Longabaugh, 1999), has been described as a primary mechanism through which recovery groups such as Alcoholics Anonymous facilitate recover (Groh, Jason, & Keys, 2007). As Chapter 9 explains in detail, the CRC is designed to provide multiple types of social support (see Salzer, 2002) to protect the abstinence of CRC members. Willis and Shinar (2000) described five types of support (emotional, validation, companionship, instrumental, and informational) that function under the umbrella of social support. The CSAR's intent is to deliver each of these to students based on their individual needs. Students' needs vary depending on age, length of recovery, and educational and family backgrounds. The CSAR provides social support through three primary paths: (a) CSAR staff, (b) peer support, and (c) referrals to other on-campus and off-campus service providers.

Despite the popularity of social support research during the past two decades, researchers have yet to establish a consistent definition of social support. According to Hutchinson (1999), definitions used in social support research should be theoretically based and operationalized according to the aims of the particular investigation. Consistent with Hutchinson's (1999) suggestion, the evaluators adapted a social support definition previously used by Cohen, Gottlieb, and Underwood (2000), defining social support provided by the CSAR as "the assistance in maintaining recovery and the protection from relapse through the provision of social resources that participants perceive to be available or that are actually provided to them in the context of Seminar and the resulting informal helping relationships established with facilitators and members." Based on the premise that prior life events and current life circumstances contribute to CSAR participants' peer-to-peer and peer-to-staff relationships, a developmental theoretical framework provides the underpinnings for the definition. The definition can be operationalized through measuring the extent to which students derive the specific types of social support from Seminar.

Emotional support. In general, emotional support is believed to be the most vital type of social support. Emotional support is demonstrated when at least one person provides concern, empathy, trust, and love to another (Krause, 1986; Langford, Bowsher, Maloney, & Lillis, 1997), resulting in feelings of esteem, attachment, and reassurance (Solomon, 2004). Emotional support is typically conveyed through sympathetic listening as one is encouraged to discuss feelings, concerns, or worries in a nonthreatening and nonjudgmental environment (Cohen et al., 2000). CRC members are thought to obtain emotional support through many settings, both in and outside of the CSAR program. These include the fellowship provided by CRC membership itself and support gained by attending conventional 12-step groups. However, possibly the most direct and structured program mechanism through which the CSAR program provides CRC members social support is through Seminar.

Validation support. Validation support is feedback that positively influences an individual's self-worth, such as affirming the appropriateness or normalcy of a person's behavior through social comparison (Willis & Shinar, 2000). This is believed to occur frequently in 12-step environments and the same dynamics are encouraged in the CRC. By observing others in recovery, recovering students are thought to have the opportunity to normalize their own recovery process, possibly lowering the stigma, shame and secrecy that often accompany addictive disorder recovery. Students can receive validation through several of the program components, such as the weekly 12-step meeting called Celebration of Recovery, often referred to as "Celebration." Celebration provides validation in three ways. First, rather than focusing on just one type of addiction, as is done at most 12-step groups; attendees at this meeting are free to express themselves about any type of addictive disorder. The meeting recognizes alcohol and other substance abuse, eating disorders, and any other addictive behaviors. The broad spectrum of addictive disorders included in Celebration places meaning on the recovery process rather than addiction, decreasing differences among various types of addictions and normalizing recovery.

Secondly, Celebration is a "birthday" meeting where group members receive "chips" that represent lengths of time in recovery. Chip recipients are congratulated and those who attend Celebration may realize that if another person can accomplish sobriety, they can too. Finally, following the distribution of birthday chips during the meeting, Celebration changes from a birthday meeting to a speaker meeting where one individual tells his or her story of recovery. Typically, this story illustrates the speaker's recovery journey and describes (a) how life was before recovery, (b) what initiated the recovery process, and (c) how recovery impacted his or her life. Hearing another person's story could normalize the addiction and recovery processes. Another CSAR program element that provides validation for recovering students is the annual holiday event that occurs during the month of December. This event is a formal gathering that spotlights the year's graduating students. Each graduate addresses a large audience filled with CSAR scholarship donors, CRC members, university administration, faculty, and staff. This graduation celebration symbolizes students' transition from college to graduate school or to the professional arena.

Companionship support. The companionship facet of social support is the construction of mutually beneficial relationships through participation in social and leisure activities (Willis & Shinar, 2000) such as going to sporting events or out to dinner. These types of activities foster a reciprocal relationship between group members who share a mutual commitment to each other (Krause, 1986). Through these relationships, individuals experience a connectedness with others and a sense of belonging. Companionship support that takes place between students in the CSAR provides a mechanism for group members to find relief from the educational aspects of college and the emotional aspects of recovery by engaging in fun and exciting activities. There are formal and informal opportunities for members to develop companionship with other group members, the most common being the informal gatherings that take place at the CSAR in between classes. Moreover, CRC members socialize together (see Chapter 6) and live together either on or off campus, also creating an atmosphere of companionship.

Instrumental support. Instrumental support includes tangible material items (food, clothes, furniture), financial help, or the provision of specific behavioral aid like transportation (Winemiller, Mitchell, Sutliff, & Cline, 1993). The main instrumental support provided by the CSAR is scholarships. The scholarships range from $500 to $2,000 per semester, depending on students' grade point averages. Often, students are drawn to the CSAR by the availability of scholarships; they may not fully realize the extent of what the CSAR has to offer. Other types of instrumental support offered at the CSAR are the new facility, tutoring (by staff and/or peers), meals at fellowship events, and class-related supplies such as scanning machines (Scantrons). The new building offers students the use of computers, study cubicles, and a large recreation room. The building is a unique commodity because it is utilized almost exclusively by recovering students, providing CSAR participants with a comfortable place to go in between classes where they can study, visit, or engage in substance-free recreational and leisure activities.

Informational support. Informational support is often provided through advice or guidance (Willis & Shinar, 2000; Solomon, 2004) that assists recipients in resolving problems (Krause, 1986; Winemiller et al., 1993; Langford et al., 1997). Informational social support also includes knowledge of where to go for other types of assistance. Although informational support provided at the CSAR is ongoing, it is given most frequently when new students join the program. At admission, students have the tasks of finding a place to live, obtaining transportation, and registering for school. If needed, CSAR Staff provides students with individualized academic advising. Staff and fellow students regularly help newer students navigate the university campus and surrounding area. Upon graduation, students may need informational support to assist them in getting through the graduation process and searching for a job.

Providing Social Support Through Seminar

In addition to staff to student contact, weekly Celebration of Recovery meetings, the fellowship of the CRC itself, the CSAR program has the unique resource provided by Seminar in Recovery. Seminar has been developed to provide a structured and consistent setting for CRC members to receive each of the social support resources detailed above. Because all CRC members are required to enroll in this specialized course each semester, it provides a potentially powerful tool to affect the recovery experience of CRC members. In fact, because the CSAR does not typically provide individual therapy to CRC members, Seminar might be considered the primary method through which the CSAR guides CRC members' recoveries. Moreover, because it is not an experience that is provided by affiliation with traditional 12-step groups it is one of the primary aspects of the CRC program that distinguishes the program from involvement in conventional 12-step groups, which is something provided or facilitated on many college and university campuses.

At the time of the evaluation, there were 11 sections of Seminar that met weekly for 1 h. Usually students are assigned to Seminar sections that correspond with their academic classification, (e.g., freshmen attend a freshmen Seminar). However, if necessary, students can be assigned to different Seminar sections to accommodate their class schedules. CSAR staff monitor Seminar enrollment to ensure that between 6 and 10 students are enrolled in any one Seminar section.

At the present time, Seminar groups are separated by gender, with the intention of increasing open and honest group discussion and providing students an opportunity to build peer-to-peer bonds between other students of the same gender. Because Seminar students receive class credit for attendance, staff members are required to submit syllabi that outline weekly topics. Usually, the topics discussed in Seminar are directly related to recovery issues or to other life skills; however, students also use this time to discuss stressful encounters that they may have experienced during that week. Seminar is uniquely geared toward recovering students by offering discussions that are specifically relevant to recovery in college contexts, such as test anxiety, peer pressure, dealing with faculty, and staying clean and sober during spring break and the winter holidays.

Method

Participants

To participate in this evaluation, students were required to be current members of the CRC and they had to attend one of two evaluation focus groups during the duration of the evaluation process. CSAR staff recruited students through email sent on behalf of the evaluators. The email stated that CRC members were being sought for an evaluation of the CSAR program and participants would be asked to complete a survey and discuss their opinions in a focus group. As an incentive, the group sessions were scheduled at meal times and pizza was served. Of the 28 students who were available during the evaluation, which took place during the summer, 14 (50%) agreed to participate in the study. Participating Seminar students were scheduled in one of two focus groups. Ten students participated in the first session and four in the second session.

Half of the 14 participants were males and all indicated their race/ethnic background as being white/non-Hispanic. Average age was $M = 24.14$ (SD = 4.0). Participants' time in recovery ranged from less than 1 to 5 years ($M = 2.79$, SD = 1.18). Number of semesters of Seminar participation ranged from one to eight ($M = 4.79$, SD = 2.08). On average, participants reported having had approximately three different staff members as Seminar facilitators over the course of their association with the program.

Measurement

A search of the literature on existing social support measurement instruments did not yield an instrument suitable to assess the five domains of social support the CSAR designed Seminar to provide. Consequently, the evaluators needed to develop an instrument to assess the extent that CRC member felt Seminar provided social support across these five domains. After participants filled out the survey instrument, they were guided through a focus group discussion about the five types of social support and asked to discuss the questions provided by the instrument, which is a process that has been found to be useful during the development of survey instruments (Klieber, 2004). The immediate goal of this instrument was to assess the effectiveness of seminar in delivering these different types of social support.

However, it is hoped that the resulting instrument could be adapted by CSAR staff to evaluate whether different aspects of the CSAR program delivers the amount and type of social support that it designed to provide. This instrument should also be useful for evaluating whether other CRC programs, whether established or newly developing, are providing similar levels and types of social support to the students in their collegiate recovery communities.

The survey, provided in Appendix, included 53 items to assess the extent to which Seminar provided students with emotional, validation, companionship, instrumental, and informational support. Students were instructed to consider the items as they pertained to their overall experience *specifically* in Seminar, but not for any particular semester. The instructions were to "circle the number that represents the extent to which you agree with the following statements." Statements were rated on a seven-point Likert scale ranging from *strongly disagree* (1) to *strongly agree* (7). Higher scores represented higher degrees of agreement.

Twelve items measured emotional support. A sample emotional support item is, "I am allowed to discuss my concerns or worries." A reverse scored sample item of emotional support item is, "Members ignore me when I discuss my problems." The survey included 11 items to measure validation support. A sample validation support item is, "I feel empowered by participating in Seminar." A reverse scored sample item of validation support item is, "I cannot identify with the members of my Seminar group." Ten items measured companionship. A sample companionship item is, "I participate in activities with members of my Seminar group away from CSAR sponsored events." A reverse scored sample item is, "I feel isolated during Seminar." Ten items were used to assess instrumental support. These included "I have received help finding, qualifying for, or applying for scholarships." A reverse scored item is, "I cannot count on someone from Seminar to provide me with the practical help I might need (such as a ride)." Because the informational domain is frequently characterized by referrals to other types of assistance, the format for the informational domain was slightly different from the other domains. Students were instructed to, "Circle the number that represents the extent to which Seminar provided you with information about the listed topics." Like the items for the four other scales, the responses ranged between 1 (strongly disagree) and 7 (strongly agree). The informational domain consisted of 10 items, including: "Academics (such as what classes to take, where to find a tutor)," and "Where to get off-campus professional services you need (such as medical, dental, counseling)." The survey also included 12 demographic questions and 5 questions about Seminar in general. As shown on Table 8.1, the subscales have acceptable Cronbach's alphas, ranging from 0.72 for emotional support to 0.89 for informational support.

Procedures. Each of the data collection meetings was organized into three phases. During the first phase, facilitators administered the survey instrument. In the second phase, they guided the participants in a focus group discussion about the instrument, asking them to comment on the clarity, comprehensiveness, relevance, as well as the potential inappropriateness or offensiveness of the survey items. In addition to the primary facilitator, two additional evaluators took notes during the sessions. The

Table 8.1 Subscale composite means (SD) and reliability $N = 14$

Subscale	Cronbach's alpha	Composite subset mean
Emotional	0.72	5.90 ($SD = 0.68$)
Validation	0.83	5.39 ($SD = 0.79$)
Companionship	0.77	5.75 ($SD = 0.78$)
Instrumental	0.82	5.41 ($SD = 1$)
Informational	0.89	5.55 ($SD = 1$)

groups were not video or audio recorded due to privacy concerns. During the third phase of the data collection meeting, the facilitator gave the group a definition of each of the five domains of social support and asked each participant to respond to two questions about how Seminar related to each domain. For example, "Does Seminar provide you with actual *informational* support when you need it?" ("Yes" or "No") and "How important is it for Seminar to provide this?" ("Very important" to "Not very important").

Results

Table 8.1 provides the means for emotional, validation, companionship, instrumental, and informational support scales. Means were used instead of sums to account for different numbers of items used to assess the five domains. All means ranged between 5.39 and 5.90. Given that the highest possible score was 7.0, these means appear to be quite high. The two types of support that were rated as most provided by Seminar were emotional (5.90) and companionship support (5.75). To the extent that there were any differences between scales, Validation (5.39) appears to be the type of support provided least by Seminar.

Validity

To consider the validity of the subscales, individual student's scores of each of the five subscales were compared to their responses to the supplemental questions about each of the five types of social support. To do this, participants' scores on subscales (e.g., emotional support) were dichotomized using a 5.0 or above (out of 7) cutoff (i.e., those above 5.0 were coded as indicating agreement that the seminar provided a high amount of that type of support. Below 5.0 were coded as not agreeing). Once coded in this way, these variables were then compared to participants' yes or no responses to the follow-up questions about whether Seminar provides that type of support when they need it. The correspondence between the dichotomously coded survey scales and the follow-up questions is shown in Table 8.2. A chi-square test of the scores from the survey and the focus groups is not significant, indicating that there were not overall differences between survey and focus group responses.

Table 8.2 Participants
confirming the functions of
seminar through survey and
focus groups ($N = 14$)

	Survey	Focus group
Emotional	13	13
Validation	11	11
Companionship	12	13
Instrumental	8	6
Informational	11	12

Given that participants responded to the follow-up questions after they were provided definitions of each social support domain, the high agreement between the
survey-derived dichotomized variables and the follow-up questions substantiates the
validity of the survey subscales.

The distributions of the scale-derived dichotomized variables and responses to
the follow-up items in Table 8.2 also highlight the differences in participants' opinions about how effectively Seminar provides different types of social support. In
contrast to the means of Table 8.2, which ranged only from 5.39 to 5.90, the
dichotomized variables and yes/no responses to the follow-up questions seem to
indicate that there were substantial systematic differences in the degree to which
Seminar provided different types of social support. For example, the responses of
13 of 14 participants were above the 5.0 cutoff in terms of whether Seminar provided emotional support. In contrast, regarding the instrumental support provided
Seminar only 8 and 6 out of 13 respondents provided responses above this threshold.
This difference suggests that although respondents have a strongly positive view of
what they get out of Seminar, there are also consistent differences between subjects
regarding which domains of support they receive more.

General Questions

In addition to the survey questions used to construct the social support scales, participants were asked to respond to several general questions regarding the importance
of Seminar to recovering students and to the recovery community. The responses to
some for these items deserve mention. For example, 12 of 14 participants (85.7%)
agreed that Seminar is important to the Collegiate Recovery Community and 10
of 14 (76.9%) indicated that they would attend even if the course were no longer
required for CRC membership. Perhaps this is because of the way Seminar is run,
as 11 out of 14 believe that the discussion format of Seminar is "just right," rather
than being too somewhat or too "fluid" or somewhat or too "rigid."

Participants were also asked to rank the seven statements about scheduling
classes and Seminar on a scale from 1, indicating most important, to 7, indicating least important. Students' rankings of the 7 statements are shown in Table 8.3
ordered by the importance participants ascribe to each statement. At the top of this
list is scheduling Seminar around other classes, allowing CSAR staff to schedule

Table 8.3 Rankings and means of the seven ways of scheduling seminar

Ranking	Mean (SD)	Aspect
1	2.57 (1.87)	I schedule Seminar around my class schedule requirements
2	3.00 (2.16)	I do not schedule my classes or Seminar, CSAR staff assists me with scheduling and I trust them to make those arrangements
3	3.62 (1.66)	I do my class and Seminar scheduling, but do not place much emphasis on the specifics of Seminar
4	4.00 (1.96)	I try to select a specific session of Seminar based on who will be members in that session
5	4.31 (1.65)	I try to select a specific session of Seminar based on who will be the facilitator
6	5.15 (1.95)	I schedule my classes around a specific session of Seminar
7	5.23 (1.64)	I select Seminar based on whether the session is/is not gender specific

Seminar, and scheduling classes without regard to specifics of Seminar. Least important for scheduling seminar were scheduling of other classes in order to enroll in a Seminar session of a specific seminar facilitator (i.e., staff or faculty member) or signing up for a specific session based on its gender composition. Thus although CRC members value Seminar generally, they do not prefer one section to another. This suggests that the perceived value of seminar is associated with the interactions of fellow CRC members and not their connection to any member of the CSAR staff. These ranking are important for two reasons. First, it appears that the different CSAR staff members who administer or oversee seminar do not change the quality, at least from the students' perspective, of the seminar experience. This is important, not only for the quality of the recovery support experience of students at TTU as the program grows there, but also for the potential replication sites. If seminar quality was dependent on one or two different staff members, and their particular skills and personalities, running Seminar sessions, this would bode poorly not only for expanding the TTU program but also for programs at other sites. These rankings are consonant with the high rankings of emotional and companionship support they associate with Seminar reported in Tables 8.1 and 8.2.

Table 8.4 provides the average scores of each of four Seminar components based on participants' ranking of each from the most to least important for them. As the order of the components indicates, participants ranked being able to freely discuss topics as needed and being able to interact with peers as more important than having

Table 8.4 Ranking and mean of the importance of the four seminar aspects

Ranking	Mean (SD)	Aspect
1	1.6 (0.76)	Freedom to discuss topics as needed
2	2.3 (1.14)	Interaction with peers
3	3 (0.88)	Section facilitator
4	3.1 (1.03)	Discussion of specific topics

either having a specific CSAR facilitator or the discussion of specific topics, which were ranked as the least important aspects of Seminar. That the ranking averages do not strongly cluster around 2.5 also indicates substantial agreement about which aspects of Seminar are the most important. Thus, students consistently perceive that the primary value of Seminar as being able to talk about topics freely and being able to talk to their student peers in recovery about them. These components map more strongly on the domains of emotional and companionship support rather than informational, instrumental, and validation support domains. It appears that CRC members value Seminar more as a supplement to their 12-step meetings than they consider it a setting to increase their knowledge of addictions. Perhaps the most important aspect of these meeting for CRC members corresponds to what conventionally aged 12 steppers get out of "normal 12-step meetings," but getting it from people who like themselves have to maintain their sobriety as young adults in the collegiate setting.

Qualitative Results

A consequence of the focus groups was the rich qualitative information gathered. The evaluators had not originally intended to consider the qualitative data beyond gaining feedback about the social support instrument. However, these discussions provided unexpected information on how CRC members view Seminar. Themes that emerged from these discussions were as follows: (a) varying meaning of Seminar according to time in recovery and as part of the CRC, (b) seminar dynamics, (c) individual characteristics, (d) scheduling, (e) and how important Seminar "is" to continued recovery.

According to students, the most important feature of Seminar is that it provides an opportunity to meet and to get to know fellow CRC members. Connections developed between students are a vital component of the community aspects of the CSAR program and it seems as if Seminar may provide the most effective way of facilitating these connections. Despite general agreement among participants that Seminar is important for their building a strong recovery, specific perceptions regarding what Seminar provides in the way of support varied by participants' time in recovery and length of involvement in the CRC. Students with less time in recovery or affiliating with the CSAR program view Seminar as being "critical" for their recovery. Students with longer lengths of time in recovery and in CSAR participation indicate Seminar as "contributing" to recovery; however, these students believe that the role of Seminar had changed for them over time (i.e. early in their Center participation, Seminar had been of greater importance).

Students indicated that several factors associated with the group dynamics within a specific section could influence the value of Seminar. For instance, female participants preferred coed sections and male participants preferred male-only sections. Group size also influenced the dynamics within sections. Larger groups limit opportunities to share with the group and decrease the confidence in the level of trust and confidentiality. Students preferred smaller groups.

Students reported that individuals' moods and personality characteristics influenced the dynamics of Seminar sections. Sometimes individuals within a Seminar section had broken confidentiality, decreasing the value of Seminar during that semester. Individuals with "dominant personalities," when left unchecked by the group facilitator, also decreased the value of the Seminar sessions. Despite not being a leading reason to schedule one seminar over another, facilitator personality, availability, and focus were mentioned frequently as affecting the value of specific sessions and semesters.

Coordinating class schedules with a desired Seminar section sometimes concerns for students. Due to schedule conflicts, some upperclassmen enrolled in freshman-level Seminar, which they did not prefer. Some students whose own recovery program was not based on the 12-step programs expressed concern about seminars being based strongly on 12-step recovery principles.

Across the board, Students believed Seminar was "critical to" or at least "contributes to" their recovery. They felt it provided a great deal of companionship and emotional support. However, informational, instrumental, and validation support was more available from other CSAR sources such as individual staff in their administrative roles, for example, talking to the associate director about scheduling or tutoring.

Discussion

The first goal of this evaluation was to create an instrument for examining the effectiveness of CSAR program components in delivering the social support they were designed to provide. The survey was administered to a small group of CRC members. Both the statistical characteristics of the social support scales (i.e., Cronbach's alphas) and concordance between dichotomized variables based on these scales and the responses to yes/no follow-up questions provide preliminary support for the reliability and validity of this new instrument.

Guided by input from CSAR staff, we focused on assessing one component of the CSAR program: The Seminar of Recovery, which staff consider one of the most, if not the most, important components of the CSAR program and is one of the elements of the CRC program at TTU that distinguishes the experience of CRC membership from being in recovery at a college or university without a CRC program. The evaluators and CSAR staff believed that assessing student perceptions of the types and amounts of social support provided by Seminar would help the CSAR more adequately understand the effectiveness of this critical program component.

As one would expect, we found some differences between staff expectations and participant perceptions. Specifically, staff believed that Seminar provided all five social support domains in largely equal amounts and, given the classroom setting as well as the presence of a CSAR staff person, if any domains of support was expected to be more evident than others they would be instrumental or informational. In contrast, both the quantitative and the qualitative data from students indicated that they perceived the social support provided by Seminar to be more strongly weighted toward the emotional and companionship domains.

Findings that students indicate that much social support is provided and that they consider it to be a valuable part of their recoveries suggest that Seminar if effective. However, it appears to work somewhat differently than the CSAR staff had expected. To establish a more realistic picture of what Seminar provides, it should be evaluated in the context of the entire CSAR program. To do this, the CSAR can modify the social support instrument presented herein to simultaneously assess the social support contributions of multiple components of the CSAR program. Such data would not only allow comparisons to be made across components, it would also allow CSAR staff to ensure that each of the 5 types of social support that the program targets were indeed being delivered. Specifically, it is important to confirm that other program components are addressing the instrumental, validation, and informational needs of the CRC members.

Measures and methods used in the present evaluation may be applied to similar programs at other universities. Specifically, the instrument provided in Appendix can be modified or similar surveys used to assess the extent to which developing programs at other colleges and universities are delivering social support across these domains. Although each program will have its own goals and methods, and input should be sought from the stakeholders in each unique program, the present findings may provide a model from which others may work when designing evaluations of their own programs.

Future Research

As this evaluation pertained to only one component of CSAR program, many questions regarding the effectiveness of the program remain, including those voiced by CSAR staff. Concerns varied substantially between staff members, ranging from how to increase the cultural diversity of the CRC to whether the rapid growth of the CSAR was decreasing the quality of services provided to CSAR students.

Another major area of concern relates the relationship between CRC and 12-step programs in general. As discussed in Chapter 2, merely referring recovering college students to 12-step programs does not adequately address their needs. But the CSAR does incorporate existing 12-step programs into its regimen. The question remains whether the CSAR should seek to increase its own programming and deemphasize its reliance on 12-step groups for providing services to CRC members. Specifically, concerns remain whether 12-step programming could address the specific developmental needs of young adults who had entered active addictions in adolescence, even where they had participated in programs directed at their needs, such as recovery high schools (Moberg & Finch, 2007). The CSAR may also wish to look more closely at the question of how to assist specific subpopulations in the community, such as students whose histories included sexual abuse.

Conclusions

In spite of the expectation that seminar would provide more instrumental or informational support than other types of social support, both the quantitative and the qualitative student reports indicated that they perceived the social support provided by Seminar to be more strongly weighted toward the emotional and companionship domains. Although the preliminary nature of this investigation requires that these results should be confirmed through further student and staff interviews, it may very well be the case that the Seminar component of the CSAR program is delivering support more emotional and companionship than instrumental or informational support. These findings do not suggest that Seminar should be changed. Rather it may be that its providing these types of support suggest it acts as an important supplement to 12-fellowship programs. Perhaps, for reasons having to do with members' age or differing viewpoints on addictions, the 12-step meetings members attend may not provide them with all the support they need. In addition, these seminars may provide a safe place that members need to form the within-community bonds that carry over to the outside of center setting of their daily lives. Consistent with this idea, perhaps the more structured (i.e., staff led) format of these meetings is a useful transition that provides familiarity to many members who have spent a lot of time "In Group" while in residential treatment. For these reasons, it seems that Seminar's ability to provide emotional and companionship support should be valued. Future research should make sure to investigate whether the instrumental or informational support Seminar is intended to provide is indeed being supplied elsewhere in necessary quantity and quality.

Appendix: CSAR Evaluation Survey Instrument

Note: Reverse Coded Statements: 13, 18, 20, 23, 25, 27, 31, 33, 35, 40, 45, 47, 51, 54.

Demographic Questionnaire

Your responses are confidential. Personal information will not be linked to your responses. Please describe yourself by filling in the blanks and circling the letters that best describe you.

1. What is your age? _____
2. What is your gender?
A. Female
B. Male
3. What is your race/ethnic background?
A. African-American/Black
B. White/Non-Hispanic
C. Hispanic/Latino
D. Native American/Alaskan Native

E. Asian/Pacific Islander

F. Other (specify) _____

4. What is your current marital status?

A. Single

B. Cohabitating

C. Engaged

D. Married/remarried

E. Life partnered

F. Divorced

G. Widowed

5. If you are a parent, do you have custody of your child?

A. Not applicable/I am not a parent

B. Yes

C. I do not have custody but I do have visitation

D. No, I don't have custody or visitation

6. When school is in session, how many hours per week do you work?

A. I do not work at all

B. 1–10 h per week

C. 11–20 h per week

D. 21–30 h per week

E. 31–40 h per week

7. What is your classification?

A. Freshman

B. Sophomore

C. Junior

D. Senior

E. Graduate Student

8. How long have you been in recovery?

A. Less than 1 year

B. 1–2 years

C. 3–5 years

D. 6–8 years

E. Over 8 years

9. How many semesters of Seminar have you taken? _____

10. How long have you participated in CSAR? _____year(s) and _____months

11. How many different Seminar facilitators have you had over the course of your participation in CSAR? _____

12. Who have been your Seminar facilitator (s)? Circle all that apply:

A. XXXXXXXXX (anonymous for this chapter)

B. XXXXXXXXX (anonymous for this chapter)

C. XXXXXXXXX (anonymous for this chapter)

   D. XXXXXXXXX (anonymous for this chapter)
   E. XXXXXXXXX (anonymous for this chapter)
   F. Others

Seminar Components Questionnaire

The following statements pertain to your overall experience *specifically* in Seminar, not a particular semester. Circle the number that represents the extent to which you agree with the following statements. Be sure to read all statements carefully.

	Strongly Disagree	Somewhat Disagree	Slightly Disagree	Neutral	Somewhat Agree	Mildly Agree	Strongly Agree
13. Members ignore me when I discuss my problems	1	2	3	4	5	6	7
14. I am allowed to discuss my concerns or worries	1	2	3	4	5	6	7
15. I am encouraged to participate in the discussion without being judged by my peers	1	2	3	4	5	6	7
16. I am encouraged to participate in the discussion without being judged by the Seminar facilitator	1	2	3	4	5	6	7
17. Seminar members appreciate my individuality and unique qualities	1	2	3	4	5	6	7

	Strongly Disagree	Somewhat Disagree	Slightly Disagree	Neutral	Somewhat Agree	Mildly Agree	Strongly Agree
18. Seminar members do not understand the emotional strain of my ongoing recovery	1	2	3	4	5	6	7
19. When I leave Seminar, I have a sense of having helped others in their recovery	1	2	3	4	5	6	7
20. Seminar makes me feel a sense of despair and pessimism	1	2	3	4	5	6	7
21. Seminar facilitators trust me to figure out my own path	1	2	3	4	5	6	7
22. Seminar members trust me to figure out my own path	1	2	3	4	5	6	7
23. Members do not understand my past experiences	1	2	3	4	5	6	7

	Strongly Disagree	Somewhat Disagree	Slightly Disagree	Neutral	Somewhat Agree	Mildly Agree	Strongly Agree
24. Seminar allows me to understand other people's recovery experiences	1	2	3	4	5	6	7
25. I receive constructive feedback on my behavior	1	2	3	4	5	6	7
26. I receive constructive feedback on my contribution to the group	1	2	3	4	5	6	7
27. I receive feedback that I have no worth or value	1	2	3	4	5	6	7
28. I receive feedback from peers in Seminar concerning my recovery process	1	2	3	4	5	6	7
29. I feel empowered by participating in Seminar	1	2	3	4	5	6	7

	Strongly Disagree	Somewhat Disagree	Slightly Disagree	Neutral	Somewhat Agree	Mildly Agree	Strongly Agree
30. Seminar facilitators provide me with encouragement that strengthens my sense of self-worth.	1	2	3	4	5	6	7
31. I cannot identify with the members of my Seminar group	1	2	3	4	5	6	7
32. I evaluate myself in light of what others say and do	1	2	3	4	5	6	7
33. I feel devalued by those in my group	1	2	3	4	5	6	7
34. I feel that I have something to offer to the Seminar group	1	2	3	4	5	6	7
35. The discussions and activities of Seminar decrease my awareness of my own ability to exercise control in my life.	1	2	3	4	5	6	7

	Strongly Disagree	Somewhat Disagree	Slightly Disagree	Neutral	Somewhat Agree	Mildly Agree	Strongly Agree
36. I participate in activities with members of my Seminar group away from CSAR sponsored events	1	2	3	4	5	6	7
37. I enjoy being with the people in Seminar	1	2	3	4	5	6	7
38. The way Seminar is conducted helps me form mutually beneficial friendships	1	2	3	4	5	6	7
39. Seminar gives me a sense of being like others	1	2	3	4	5	6	7
40. I feel isolated during Seminar	1	2	3	4	5	6	7
41. Seminar allows me to meet others who support me in my daily progress	1	2	3	4	5	6	7

	Strongly Disagree	Somewhat Disagree	Slightly Disagree	Neutral	Somewhat Agree	Mildly Agree	Strongly Agree
42. Seminar has helped me to reconsider the meanings of past, current, and future relationships	1	2	3	4	5	6	7
43. My determination to maintain recovery has increased because Seminar provides me with friends who are successful in recovery	1	2	3	4	5	6	7
44. Seminar allows me to meet others who value my recovery efforts	1	2	3	4	5	6	7
45. I seldom get invited to do things with others from Seminar	1	2	3	4	5	6	7
46. I have received help finding, qualifying for, or applying for scholarships	1	2	3	4	5	6	7

	Strongly Disagree	Somewhat Disagree	Slightly Disagree	Neutral	Somewhat Agree	Mildly Agree	Strongly Agree
47. I have received little to no help making appointments for services within the community in Seminar	1	2	3	4	5	6	7
48. I have the opportunity to provide practical help (such as a ride) to other Seminar members	1	2	3	4	5	6	7
49. Seminar provides me with the opportunity to practice life skills (such as time management)	1	2	3	4	5	6	7
50. I have received handouts or other written information that have been useful to me	1	2	3	4	5	6	7

	Strongly Disagree	Somewhat Disagree	Slightly Disagree	Neutral	Somewhat Agree	Mildly Agree	Strongly Agree
51. I cannot count on someone from Seminar to provide me with the practical help I might need (such as a ride)	1	2	3	4	5	6	7
52. Seminar participation provides me with skills to aid my recovery process	1	2	3	4	5	6	7
53. Seminar participation provides me with skills to help me succeed as a student	1	2	3	4	5	6	7
54. Seminar participation does not provide me with skills that prepare me for life after graduation	1	2	3	4	5	6	7

	Strongly Disagree	Somewhat Disagree	Slightly Disagree	Neutral	Somewhat Agree	Mildly Agree	Strongly Agree
	1	2	3	4	5	6	7
55. I receive reminders that my words of support or encouragement are helpful to other Seminar members							

The following statements pertain to your overall experience *specifically* in Seminar, not a particular semester. Circle the number that represents the extent to *which Seminar provided you with information about the listed topics.*

	Strongly Disagree	Somewhat Disagree	Slightly Disagree	Neutral	Somewhat Agree	Mildly Agree	Strongly Agree
56. Academics (such as what classes to take, where to find a tutor)	1	2	3	4	5	6	7
57. Addiction issues	1	2	3	4	5	6	7
58. Coping with life's problems, stressors, and hassles	1	2	3	4	5	6	7
59. How to get along with your peers	1	2	3	4	5	6	7
60. How to access on-campus student services	1	2	3	4	5	6	7
61. Careers services (such as career counseling, job placement)	1	2	3	4	5	6	7

	Strongly Disagree	Somewhat Disagree	Slightly Disagree	Neutral	Somewhat Agree	Mildly Agree	Strongly Agree
62. Where to get off-campus professional services you need (such as medical, dental, counseling)	1	2	3	4	5	6	7
63. The recovery process	1	2	3	4	5	6	7
64. Services CSAR provides	1	2	3	4	5	6	7
65. Creating a supportive recovery network when away from CSAR (such as during holidays, after graduation)	1	2	3	4	5	6	7

General Seminar Questionnaire

66. Seminar is important to the recovery community of CSAR
    A. Yes
    B. No

67. If Seminar were no longer a requirement of participation with CSAR, I would continue to attend
    A. Agree
    B. Disagree

68. Circle the letter which corresponds with how you would complete the following sentence:
    I feel the discussion format of Seminar is:
    A. Too Rigid
    B. Somewhat rigid
    C. Just Right
    D. Somewhat Fluid
    E. Too Fluid

69. What aspect of Seminar is most important to you?
    Rank in order of importance, with (1) as most important and (4) as least important:
    ———Facilitator
    ———Interaction with peer group
    ———Discussions of specific topics
    ———Freedom to discuss topics as the need arises

70. Rank the following statements regarding scheduling classes and Seminar, with (1) as most important and (7) as least important:
    In scheduling Seminar:
    ———I schedule my classes around a specific session of Seminar
    ———I schedule Seminar around my class schedule requirements
    ———I try to select a specific session of Seminar based on who will be members in that session
    ———I try to select a specific session of Seminar based on who will be the facilitator
    ———I do my class and Seminar scheduling, but do not place much emphasis on the specifics of Seminar
    ———I do not schedule my classes or Seminar, CSAR staff assists me with scheduling and I trust them to make those arrangements
    ———I select Seminar based on whether the session is/is not gender specific

References

Beattie, M., & Longabaugh, R. (1999). General and alcohol-specific social support following treatment. *Addictive Behaviors, 24,* 593–606.
Cohen, S., Gottlieb, B. H., & Underwood, L. G. (2000). Social relationships and health. In S. Cohen, L. G. Underwood, & B. H. Gottlieb (Eds.), *Social support measurement and intervention* (pp. 3–25). New York: Oxford University Press.

Groh, D. B., Jason, L. A., & Keys, C. B. (2007). Social network variables in alcoholics anonymous: A literature review. *Clinical Psychology Review*, *28*, 430–450.

Hutchinson, C. (1999). Social support: Factors to consider when designing studies that measure social support. *Journal of Advanced Nursing*, 29, 1520–1526.

Klieber, P. B. (2004). Focus groups: More than a method of qualitative inquiry. In K. de Marris & S. Lapan (Eds.), *Foundations for research: Methods of inquiry in education and the social sciences* (pp. 87–102). Mahwah, NJ: L. Eribaurm Associates.

Krause, N. (1986). Social support, stress, and well-being among older adults. *Journal of Gerontology*, 41, 512–519.

Langford, C. P. H., Bowsher, J., Maloney, J. P., & Lillis, P. P. (1997). Social support: A conceptual analysis. *Journal of Advanced Nursing*, 25, 95–100.

Moberg, D., & Finch, A. (2007). Recovery high schools as continuing care for substance use disorders. *Journal of Groups in Addiction & Recovery*, 2, 128–161.

Salzer, M. S. (2002). *Best practice guidelines for consumer-delivered services*. Peoria, IL: Behavioral Health Recovery Management Project; Bloomington, IL: Chestnut Health Systems.

Solomon, P. (2004). Peer support/peer provided services underlying processes, benefits, and critical ingredients. *Psychiatric Rehabilitation Journal*, 27, 392–401.

Willis, T. A., & Shinar, O. (2000). Measuring perceived and received social support. In S. Cohen, L. G. Underwood, & B. H. Gottlieb (Eds.), *Social support measurement and intervention* (pp. 86–135). New York: Oxford University Press.

Winemiller, D. R., Mitchell, M. E., Sutliff, J., & Cline, D. J. (1993). Measurement strategies in social support: A descriptive review of the literature. *Journal of Clinical Psychology*, 5, 638–648.

Chapter 9
Establishing College-Based Recovery Communities: Opportunities and Challenges Encountered

Amanda Baker

Persons aged 18–25 have among the highest rates of alcohol and illicit drug abuse and dependence in the nation (Substance Abuse and Mental Health Services Administration, 2008), creating significant challenges to American colleges and universities. In response, these institutions have poured and will continue to pour millions of dollars into student health and service programs aimed at combating what has been labeled by some as an substance abuse epidemic (Wechsler & Weuthrich, 2002). Most programs have focused on primary and secondary prevention efforts such as social norming, alcohol- and drug-free social activities, risk reduction (i.e., safe ride home programs), and the development and enforcement of zero tolerance policies. Despite these efforts at prevention, young adulthood continues to be the most common developmental period for the onset of alcohol and drug use disorders (Caldeira et al., 2009). From 1998 to 2005, colleges have seen increases in heavy episodic drinking, driving under the influence of alcohol, and rates of unintentional alcohol-related nontraffic injury deaths (Hingson, Zha, & Weitzman, 2009). Likewise, the number of students who reported being physically or sexually assaulted by another student under the influence of alcohol or drugs or who reported injury by themselves due to being under the influence of alcohol remained high. The most current governmental reporting provides that 18- to 25-year-olds make up almost one-quarter (22%) of treatment admissions in the United States (SAMHSA, 2008).

Somewhere between 6% (Wechsler & Weuthrich, 2002) and 25% (The National Center on Addiction and Substance Abuse at Columbia University, 2007) of college students exhibit symptoms that would qualify them for alcohol and/or drug dependency disorders according to established clinical criteria. The standard prevention efforts used by colleges and universities do not address the needs of the growing number of young college students who are either trying to become abstinent or trying to maintain hard-won abstinence from alcohol and other drugs. Instead, these students need abstinence-focused community support. Though some college

A. Baker (✉)
Texas Tech University, Lubbock, TX, USA
e-mail: amanda.k.baker@ttu.edu

H.H. Cleveland et al. (eds.), *Substance Abuse Recovery in College*, Advancing
Responsible Adolescent Development, DOI 10.1007/978-1-4419-1767-6_9,
© Springer Science+Business Media, LLC 2010

and university campuses have implemented identification, intervention, and referral plans for individual students needing treatment, few have taken steps to safeguard the abstinence of students returning to campus after treatment or have considered the needs of students who start their college careers in recovery from an addictive disorder. Apart from providing access to traditional 12-step approaches, which may have limits when used as the sole means of recovery support for college-aged individuals (Harrison & Hoffmann, 1987; Kelly & Myers, 2007), campuses rarely provide services for their recovering student populations.

As is made clear by other chapters in this volume, establishing college-based recovery communities is one way colleges and universities can support and ultimately retain students who have substance use issues and who would like to pursue recovery from their addictive disorder, whether such dependency develop prior to or during their enrollment. This chapter describes the efforts made by the Texas Tech University (TTU) Center for the Study of Addiction and Recovery (CSAR) to document the TTU Collegiate Recovery Community (CRC) program and export it to other colleges and universities. In addition, it provides specific details about the CSAR's work with three institutions of higher learning, as each begins to build their own college recovery community program.

Documenting the CRC Model: Building Theory Around Experience

Between 1997and 2008, the CRC at TTU grew from 20 to 75 members, as applications increased from around 10 to over 50 per year. This increase in size coincided with the realization that current CRC members were thriving, in terms of both maintaining abstinence in the college environment and succeeding academically. As the CRC's success was becoming apparent, the CSAR was motivated to encourage and assist other colleges and universities in developing similar programs. Initial efforts, supported through the first of two congressionally directed grants, focused on placing the service components of the CRC program into a unified model that emphasizes the role of peer-based social support in initiating and maintaining positive lifestyle changes among those in recovery. Using this model as a catalyst, the CSAR developed a curriculum designed to guide other colleges/universities in the process of developing recovery support communities. A copy of the full curriculum (Harris, Baker, & Thompson, 2005) may be obtained directly from the CSAR.

When the CSAR set out to develop its comprehensive curriculum, however, we faced some challenges. The first was that that college-based recovery programs, including the one at Texas Tech, had evolved over time instead of resting on a single dominant theoretical foundation. This meant that we had to discover and formally articulate whatever theory might be embedded in these programs including its own. Unfortunately, college recovery communities, though nearly three decades old at the time, had not generated much formal research to aid in this process of discovery. College-based recovery programs began in 1977, with the first one at

Brown University (White & Finch, 2006), and developed mostly independently of one another over the next three decades. At the time of this writing, approximately 12 CRC programs exist in the United States, most of which were developed in 1999 or later; a current list can be found at the Association of Recovery Schools website, www.recoveryschools.org.

Apart from internally generated marketing and public relations materials, these programs are not very well-documented. Two reasons for this lack of documentation are as follows: first, most programs serve relatively few students (see Chapter 2 for a review of program models), making it difficult to statistically analyze either program process or program effect, and second, their isolation from each other, at least until the formation of the Association of Recovery Schools in 2002. Because of the importance of the problem—the paucity of recovery programs on American campuses—we felt we could not afford to wait for mature research in the area and pursued a grounded theory approach in order to provide a solid theoretical base for its "how-to" curriculum.

As the first step in this process, CSAR staff surveyed marketing materials of existing college-based recovery programs, visited sites, and interviewed participating staff and students. Only programs that had been open for more than 5 years were included in this information-gathering phase.

Three common elements emerged from this phase, each of which revolved around the central issue of social support (see Chapter 6 and Chapter 8). First, the recovery communities themselves seemed to need support from their larger college and university communities. The degree of success of college-based recovery communities appeared to be tied to the extent of commitment and support (i.e., "buy-in") they received from campus entities, including the college or university administration, campus-based mental health providers, and faculty, staff, and students in recovery.

Second, community members appeared to receive their key support from the community itself. Thus, it appears that in a successful community, the primary source of recovery support comes from membership in a community wherein individual students both give and receive assistance. This kind of abstinent-specific social support (Beattie & Longabaugh, 1999; see Chapter 7) ranges beyond what well-meaning, relatively sober, friends and family can provide and seems especially important in a college environment soaked with intoxicating substances.

Third, college-based recovery communities were not merely 12-step programs conducted on campus. Instead, they went beyond the 12-step model in two significant ways: They integrated professional service with peer support and they addressed education as well as recovery. The message seems to be that a college administration that merely provided students with a list of nearby AA and NA meetings would not be doing enough.

All of these commonalities reflected the importance of social support. With them in mind, the CSAR began to focus on finding and applying a framework to help us consider how these communities aid the continued recovery of their members in terms of social support. We found such a framework in the peer-based social support paradigm proposed by Salzer (2002). This social support typology was developed to evaluate psychiatric rehabilitation programs, but has proven beneficial for developing the language and methods of inquiry used to describe and study recovery communities both inside and outside of higher education.

Salzer describes five domains of peer-driven social support: (1) emotional support, (2) informational support, (3) instrumental support, (4) validation, and (5) companionship (1997). In order to assist their membership in both initiating and sustaining positive lifestyle change in both recovery- and academic-related tasks, we believe that communities must provide access to peer-driven social support across each of these five domains. That support exist across all these domains is critical. While many campuses offer individual services that address one or two domains of social support (i.e., 12-step meetings, individual and/or group counseling, and cohort specific academic advising), these components alone do not provide a comprehensive environment in which individual recovering students can sustain their recoveries and nurture their academic success. Thus, it is only by providing services that both address and interweave each of the five types of social support that universities and colleges can ensure their CRC programs adequately protect both the recovery and educational goals of students within them.

Below we consider how collegiate recovery communities focus on supporting the recovery and educational needs of their members through these five domains of social support.

Emotional support. The first domain is emotional support, which is defined as demonstrations of empathy, love, caring, and concern. The existence of sufficient emotional support depends on the expression of shared joy and pain between individuals who have experienced common life events. To ensure that members are receiving the emotional support needed, CRC programs focus on harnessing "the power of interaction between those with similar or shared experiences" and using this power to facilitate change (Salzer, 2002). In the context of CRC programs, this type of support manifests under the linked umbrellas of peer and recovering professional mentoring, as well as interpersonal exchanges during recovery support group meeting (see also Chapter 8). Unlike program components that deliver companionship support, emotional support involves both interactions between students in recovery and other students and interactions between recovering students and professional staff members. That professional staff members are involved in this domain of support underscores a critical difference between a college- or university-sponsored recovery program and a freestanding 12-step community that, in essence, happens to be comprised of students.

Informational support. The second domain of peer-driven social support is informational support. Informational support is defined as advice or guidance to assist with problem-solving and evaluation for choosing between alternative actions to deal with a given problem. In addition, informational support often provides recovering individuals with health and wellness information, educational assistance, and help in acquiring new skills, ranging from life skills to employment readiness. Due to their histories of being disconnected from secondary education, students with addictions have a heightened need for informational support. Moreover, as Chapter 3 emphasizes, adolescence is normatively a time during which individuals develop their methods of coping with life events and formulate the skills, competencies, and goals that they will use in young adulthood (Cote, 2000; Erikson, 1968). The interference of alcoholism and drug addiction with the development of problem-solving and behavioral skills, especially as these skills address interactions with social institutions, can have lasting effects individuals whose addiction took hold during adolescence (Chapter 3 by Russell et al., this volume). Many individuals who join CRC programs began their substance use behaviors at very young ages. As a result, not only do they need to determine who they are as young adults without the benefit of sober adolescent life experiences, but in many cases they must learn basic problem-solving and self-care skills needed to successfully pursue academic and professional goals. By providing informational support, CRC programs can help recovering young adults begin to acquire these basic coping skills and competencies.

Instrumental support. The third domain of support is instrumental. This type of support involves assisting recovering individuals with navigating societal systems. This form of social support often involves concrete assistance in task accomplishment, especially with stressful or unpleasant tasks such as filling out applications, finding child care, and locating means of transportation for people in recovery to support-group meetings. Unfortunately, active addiction often exhausts the instrumental support systems of the afflicted individuals and families. Thus, by the time addicts enter recovery and may be able to use any instrumental support provided to them, the systems that could deliver it are exhausted. Without instrumental support, the risk of relapse increases.

One of the goals of the CRC, therefore, is to provide a new source of instrumental support that is specifically tailored to the needs of recovering young adults pursuing their educations. Different college-based recovery programs provide this instrumental support in different ways. The TTU CRC program provides scholarships to recovering students to help offset the cost of education and housing. Other programs provide instrumental support by offering designated recovery housing (see Chapter 2).

Validation support. The fourth domain of support that college-based recovery programs need to provide is validation support. This type of support centers on the principle of social comparison. Validation results from the belief that one's actions and behaviors are appropriate or normal when compared with those of peers (Willis & Shinar, 2000). Recovering students engage in behaviors, such as attending 12-step meetings, praying or meditating, and abstaining from drugs and alcohol, which seem non-normative for a typical college student. As a result, recovering students are at risk for making negative self-evaluations if they use their nonrecovering peers as their primary reference group. College-based recovery communities provide recovering students with alternate reference groups that increase the likelihood of positive social comparisons and help them establish a social identity that facilitates recovery (see Lennon, Gallois, Owen, & McDermott, 2005). If recovery students see that they are similar in thought and action to a group of their peers, recovery behaviors are reinforced and social stigma is reduced or eliminated resulting in validation. Examples of CRC program components that promote validation at TTU include Celebration of Recovery meetings and Seminar classes (see also Chapter 8).

Companionship support. The fifth domain of social support is companionship support. This type of support addresses an acute challenge for students in recovery: The difficulty of resisting social pressures toward "group conformity in an alcohol-saturated environment" (Perkins, 2002, p. 166). Companionship with others in recovery can help people in recovery feel connected and enjoy being with others, especially during substance-free recreational activities. While college-based recovery programs do not seek to isolate members from the college culture, reinforcing abstinence through peer relationships and giving members a respite from social triggers and peer pressures to use substances are critical. This assistance is especially needed in early recovery, when little about abstaining from alcohol or drugs is easy. Companionship social support, more that other types of social support, depends on a strong network of abstinent peers. For this support to function, recovering students must provide and accept social support from their community.

Documenting "Real Life" Experience

Equally important to establishing a theory-based model of CRC programming is addressing issues that involve the start-up, administration, and evaluation of a recovery support program. Although the social networks of fellow recovering young persons provide the primary ingredient for continuing abstinence, communities require administrative support. Unfortunately, not all colleges and universities have staff in a position to work with a recovery program who have personal experience with recovery. Potential administrators need information and training on how different social support mechanisms enact positive lifestyle change for people in recovery.

To identify the "real life" logistics of implementing the CRC model, CSAR staff identified specific content areas they believed warranted inclusion in the final curriculum. Content areas were then organized into four categories corresponding to "projects," to be implemented sequentially when establishing a college-based recovery community. The result is a comprehensive document that explains the process of creating such a community from start to finish, a process estimated to take 1 year. The following sections provide an overview of the suggested steps for developing and implementing recovery communities on college and university campuses.

Project One: Moving Ideas into Action

Professionals and paraprofessionals associated with substance abuse prevention have used community coalition building as an effective method for disseminating new ideas and building support for innovative, community-based programs (Flewelling et al., 2005). Likewise, start-up programs can use this approach to transform the idea of recovery support services into a viable proposal for administrators. In the course of Project One, program supporters begin by "organizing a Project Planning Team and moving through the basic groundwork of strategic planning, fundraising, and gaining administrative support for [a] Collegiate

Recovery Community" (Harris et al., 2005, p. 7). Before proposing a CRC-type program at a college or university, advocates should know which and how many students the program will serve, how much it will cost and where the funding will come from, and which administrative unit will maintain administrative responsibility for program personnel and operations. Some of the most common barriers to accessing administrative support for CRC programs include (a) the view that recovering students are a liability rather than an asset to the campus, (b) a scarcity of financial resources and space for start-up programs, (c) the idea that the student population served by recovery communities will be too small to benefit the campus as a whole, and (d) the fear that CRC programs could take resources away from campus counseling centers and/or clinics (Harris et al., 2005).

Project Two: Organizing and Implementing Social Support Components

Assessing existing campus services is one of the most crucial steps in creating CRC programs. Many campuses offer some of the social support components needed to create a recovery community, though these components are not often organized into a comprehensive support program for recovering students. Rather, they operate independently of one another and fail to create the social support mechanisms required by the CRC model. Project Two focuses on planning how recovery-specific programming can be developed to integrate with existing services to create a new recovery support service on college and university campuses.

Plans for integrating these components must recognize that the needs of recovering students will vary across campus communities, depending on both student and campus characteristics. If social support interventions are to be effective, services must include a mix of peer- and staff-delivered services. For example, 12-step meetings are solely peer-based, since recovering individuals and only recovering individuals interact with one another to provide support for recovery. In contrast to a program that relies solely on 12-step traditions, the CSAR model requires interactions between recovering student and professional members of the college or university staff, such as counselors and academic advisors. One of the most important tasks of Project Two is to address the balance between the traditional 12-step peer-only support system and the university's or college's professional support system in providing the various types of social support described above. The CSAR curriculum (Harris et al., 2005) details methods of multiple activities that have proven successful in different college-based recovery programs.

Project Three: Operations and Administration

Program design and community support are the building blocks of CRC programs. However, effective handling of daily operational tasks and personnel issues is essential for the success of a program. Currently, college-based recovery communities can be found in three different organizational units within the college/university system: academic departments (e.g., the CSAR is housed in the College of Human Sciences), student health services, and student services/campus life. Each of these organizational units possesses assets and liabilities for implementing and maintaining CRC programs. However, regardless of where the recovery community is based, it will face several operational challenges, including, but not limited to, (a) student recruitment and referral, (b) staffing patterns, (c) advisory boards and fundraising teams, and (d) membership application review.

Project Four: Program Evaluation

Literature addressing the outcomes and effectiveness of CRC programs is scant. As of early 2009, only two of the existing CRC programs, the CSAR at Texas Tech and the StepUp Program at Augsburg College, had data collection and analysis measures in place and no fully fledged implementation or outcome evaluations of any college-based recovery program had been published or even completed. As a result, the recovery literature seldom even mentions college-based recovery communities and, for the most part, CRC-type programs have been unsuccessful in securing research funding.

Project Four emphasizes the importance of program evaluation and suggests strategies and tools to measure program success, focusing more on formative evaluation—e.g., obtaining and documenting stakeholder (i.e., CRC staff/faculty, college/university administration, recovering students) feedback during the implementation process—than on summative or outcome evaluation. It does recommend, however, that CRC programs at the minimum keep records of three relevant outcome variables from the beginning: (a) relapse rate, (b) GPA of enrolled students, and (c) retention rate of students and reasons for withdrawal from the program.

Pilot Programs: Exporting CRC Programs to Other Campuses

Once the CSAR had completed its initial work on a comprehensive curriculum for creating a college-based recovery community (Harris et al., 2005), we subjected the curriculum to a series of content reviews and revisions by two independent evaluator panels, from both within and outside TTU, consisting of university administrators; mental health professionals, some of who had experience working in CRC-type programs; and members of recovery communities. Beyond providing substantive feedback on the curriculum, the evaluator panels recommended that CSAR staff conduct three pilot trials of the curriculum. Pilot trials were to serve two purposes: First, to determine the effectiveness of the existing curriculum documentation for assisting other colleges and universities in implementing CRC programs on their campuses and second, to provide feedback from pilot implementation sites regarding the challenges that different campuses can encounter when attempting to establish their own recovery communities.

Selection of Pilot Sites

The first step in implementing the evaluators' recommendation was to select the pilot sites. During the first year of replication work, the CSAR was contacted by representatives from numerous entities interested in becoming pilot sites for CRC replication programs. These contacts included eight different colleges and universities—four research-oriented universities, one liberal arts college, and three community colleges—from four different states; two government representatives, and two private substance abuse treatment facilities. Since the CSAR's primary intent is to develop recovery support mechanisms within higher education contexts, government agencies and private treatment facilities were not considered as potential pilot sites.

Each of the interested colleges and universities was asked to provide the following information: (a) evidence of accreditation as an institution of higher education; (b) a memorandum from a counseling center or therapy clinic agreeing to provide services for any recovering students participating in a CRC program, even if the CRC program ceased to exist on that campus; (c) the name of a contact person currently employed by the institution; and (d) a letter stating that the institution agreed to allow representatives of the CSAR access to participating faculty, staff, and students for up to 2 years from the beginning of the collaborative relationship for the purposes of collecting data to further develop the CRC replication model. Only five of the eight interested institutions provided the requested documentation.

Description of Pilot Sites

To narrow the list to the final three, we considered student demographics and the proposed location of the CRC program within the administrative structure. The goal was to choose the three most divergent institutions—from Texas Tech as well as from each other—to enhance external reliability.

Demographic factors included the number, age, and racial/ethnic makeup of enrolled students, and the number of enrolled students who resided in on-campus housing. Additionally, the CSAR chose pilot sites that intended to locate their CRC programs in varying administrative locations within the campus structure.

The first pilot site chosen was a large university in the Mountain West region of the United States, which showed remarkable similarity to TTU in all demographic factors, but opted to house its CRC program in the Division of Student Affairs.

The second pilot site was a large university in the Southwest with a comparable sized student enrollment, but served a primarily Hispanic population. This university site is more of a commuter campus than either TTU or the Mountain West pilot university. At this site, the pilot program was to be administratively nested in Student Counseling Services.

The third site is a four-campus community college system. Currently, it is one of only two community college systems nationwide to maintain a recovery community on campus, and is the only institution that maintains a CRC-type program in a multi-campus format. Its recovery community is housed in an academic department. This institution is also in the Southwest. Unlike TTU, it serves primarily nontraditional students (i.e., those over the age of 25).

Working Collaboratively Across Institutions

As noted above, to design, develop, and implement the beginnings of CRC program requires about a year. Thus, collaborative relationships between the CSAR and pilot sites ran from the beginning of the grant funding cycle (July 2005) until its close (July 2006). During this year, representatives of the CSAR visited each site at least twice, and each pilot site sent two representatives from its campus to TTU for a 4-day training session. Pilot sites had immediate access to CRC model curriculum documents prior to final publication and were asked to provide feedback on the content and organization of these materials, as they related to their attempts to implement a CRC program on their campus. For additional technical assistance support, all pilot sites maintained contact with CSAR staff through telephone and email correspondence, and have continued to do so, using internal funding resources, even after the formal, funded collaboration period ended in July of 2006.

A key component of working with different pilot sites was understanding the needs of each site. At the beginning of the collaboration process, questionnaires were used to assess the knowledge of each pilot site's program leaders in areas related to CRC programs. Questions covered topics such as recovery and college life, grant writing/fundraising, administration/staffing, student recruitment, and program assessment. In addition, pilot site leaders were asked to document specific obstacles they anticipated or problems they had already encountered in developing CRC programs on their campuses. The questionnaire provided CSAR staff with information about specific campus challenges that might be encountered and allowed staff to design consulting plans and approaches for each replication site. It further informed the content of the final CRC program curriculum by (1) outlining the strengths and weaknesses in the knowledge base of college/university representatives who would be potential CRC program directors, (2) documenting anticipated obstacles in program implementation and maintenance of three unique campuses, and (3) providing feedback on topics that CSAR staff may have overlooked when determining curriculum content. Although the information from three pilot sites cannot be generalized to all institutions of higher education, feedback from these initial collaborations offers insight about the types of challenges that can be encountered when implementing CRC programs across different university settings.

Identified Challenges

Implementing the CRC model in a diverse array of college campuses presented challenges for both CSAR staff and pilot institution representatives. Predictably, those challenges centered around funding and staffing issues.

Funding. In early stages of documenting the CRC model, we found that existing programs' annual operating budgets ranged substantially from as low as $40,000 to as high as $250,000 with larger and older programs having the largest budgets. From interviews and historical budget records provided by existing college-based recovery community program directors, it is estimated that a new CRC-type program needs $50,000–$100,000 annually to offer comprehensive recovery support services that include all five types of social support from paying staff salaries to funding student scholarships and purchasing coffee.

Regardless of the size of their proposed budgets, pilot programs had difficulty accessing the required funding for their programs. In each case, the initial source approached for funding was the university. While each pilot program received some financial support from their home institution, the amount was inadequate to fully fund a comprehensive CRC at any pilot site. Reasons cited by the university for not fully funding the program included that (a) the program would not serve a broad enough population or a large enough number of students, (b) because little documented evidence exists to demonstrate the success of this model, it should only be funded at the level of an exploratory program, and (c) the program would be so specialized that it was unclear which department, division, or college should house it, so it was also unclear as to who should fund it.

Pilot site personnel also experienced difficulty in securing dollars from grant awards at the state or federal levels. Although their goal may be seen as relapse prevention, college-based recovery communities are often not seen by government funding agencies as falling into the traditional divisions of the substance abuse prevention or treatment. Nor do they seem to fail under fundable areas of bio-behavioral research or pharmacology. This results in few competitive funding opportunities for which CRC programs would meet eligibility criteria. Though pilot sites reported looking actively at various requests for proposals, not one site was successful in securing competitive grant or contract dollars from a government funding agency. In view of the experiences of existing college recovery communities, this result was not surprising. While some extant programs have received federal funding through the earmarking process or through agency discretionary funding, competitive dollars have been difficult to access.

In contrast, pilot programs did report success in securing funds from the private sector through individual donations and through private foundation awards. Program directors reported gifts from $50 to $100,000 with the majority of the funds classified as unrestricted and therefore available for the program to use in any needed area. Again, this comported with the experiences of extant programs. Seeking funding from private donors and foundations has proven to be more successful than attempting to pursue funding within the university system or from public agencies.

Staffing. The CSAR consulting plan and replication curriculum recommends that a new CRC program begin operations with a minimum of two staff members: A program director and an administrative coordinator. Limited resources prevented any of the pilot sites from opening with this staffing structure. Two opened with a part-time (20 h per week) commitment and one opened with a full-time commitment allocated between two people. Pilot program staff reported that it was difficult to fulfill the responsibilities associated with the CRC program in 20 h per week. Specifically, staff reported that fundraising, student recruitment, and responding to telephone and email inquiries about the program were the three responsibilities most likely to be left uncompleted. Meeting with recovering students, completing reports for administration/job supervisors, and marketing of community-based program were the responsibilities most likely to be completed.

Pilot program staff also reported that the mix of administrative and student services/counseling duties was difficult to navigate. Many of the individuals selected as program directors and staff had experience in one area or the other, but none reported feeling equally competent in both areas. For strong administrators, the level of student interaction and support provision was reported to be difficult, especially for staff with little experience working with a recovering population. In contrast, the program directors and staff who excelled at providing student services and support found that both fundraising and interacting with upper-level administrators were intimidating.

Conclusions

Of the three pilot programs, two are still operating at this writing. The third pilot program was eliminated due to a change in administrative priorities for student services programs. At its closing, it had been providing recovery support services to 20 students.

Apparently as a result of the piloting process reported here, five additional schools have implemented recovery support services on their campus using the TTU CRC model as a template. The net result is that there are seven more college-based recovery communities based on the CSAR curriculum than there were when the CSAR was first funded for this purpose in 2004. It is estimated that the opening of these programs have provided additional support for 200 recovering students across the country.

Clearly, it is good to have a theory of recovery and a curriculum in place, but many administrators and funding agencies will remain skeptical until they can see strong evidence that college-based recovery can work. In this volume, we have presented information regarding the high academic achievement and low relapse rates of CRC members at TTU (see Chapter 4), but clearly more program evaluation research should be performed. Toward this end, in the spring of 2009, the eight institutions with TTU-based CRC programs participated in the founding meeting of the Collegiate Recovery Community Research Consortium. The goal of this new consortium is to develop and implement measures to quantify the impact of these programs on both individuals in recovery and their campuses and institutions. Current feedback from program directors of CRC programs across the country regarding relapse rates, GPAs, and graduations, has been encouraging, strongly suggesting that students are staying in recovery, excelling academically, and graduating to post-college lives with strong recoveries and bright futures.

The CSAR program has evolved over two decades to promote recovery and to make education accessible for the growing numbers of young adults in recovery from alcohol and drugs, based on a theory that uses a comprehensive array of social support (Salzer, 2002) to promote healthy individual (Erikson, 1968) and social (Lennon et al., 2005) identity development. By providing social support in otherwise abstinence-hostile environments, colleges and universities across the country can use the CSAR model to aid many more recovering students than are currently being served. According to the directors of new and established college-based recovery programs, student participation in these communities is increasing. As more colleges and universities implement recovery support programs and information about how to successfully implement these programs is refined, evidence will accumulate regarding the effectiveness of these programs. If the effectiveness of these programs can be empirically established, it is hoped that they can be implemented on a widespread basis.

References

Beattie, M., & Longabaugh, R. (1999). General and alcohol-specific social support following treatment. *Addictive Behaviors, 24,* 593–606.

Caldeira, K. M., Kasperski, S. J., Sharma, E., Vincent, K. B., O'Grady, K. E., Wish, E. D., et al. (2009). College students rarely seek help despite serious substance use problems. *Journal of Substance Abuse Treatment* (in press).

Cote, J. E. (2000). *Arrested adulthood: The changing nature of maturity and identity*. New York: NYU Press.

Erikson, E. H. (1968). *Identity: Youth and crisis*. New York: Norton & Company.

Flewelling, R. L., Austin, D., Hale, K., LaPlante, M., Liebig, M., Piasecki, L., et al. (2005). Implementing research-based substance abuse prevention in communities: Effects of a coalition-based prevention initiative in Vermont. *Journal of Community Psychology, 33,* 333–353.

Harris, K. S., Baker, A. K., & Thompson, A. A. (2005). *Making an opportunity for your campus: A comprehensive curriculum for designing a collegiate recovery community*. Washington, DC: Substance Abuse and Mental Health Services Administration and the US Department of Education.

Harrison, P. A., & Hoffmann, N. G. (1987). *CATOR report: Adolescent residential treatment, intake and follow-up findings*. St. Paul, MN: Ramsey Clinic.

Hingson, R. W., Zha, W., & Weitzman, E. R. (2009). Magnitude of and trends in alcohol-related mortality and morbidity among US college students ages 18–25, 1998–2005. *Journal of Studies on Alcohol and Drugs, 16,* 12–20.

Kelly, J. F., & Myers, M. G. (2007). Adolescent's participation in Alcoholics Anonymous and Narcotics Anonymous: Review, implications, and future directions. *Journal of Psychoactive Drugs, 39,* 259–269.

Lennon, A., Gallois, C., Owen, N., & McDermott, L. (2005). Young women as smokers and nonsmokers: A qualitative social identity approach. *Qualitative Health Research, 15*, 1345–1359.

National Center on Addiction and Substance Abuse at Columbia University. (2007). *Wasting the best and the brightest: Substance abuse at America's colleges and universities.*

Perkins, H. W. (2002). Social norms and the prevention of alcohol misuse in collegiate contexts. *Journal of Studies on Alcohol, 14*, 164–172.

Salzer, M. S. (2002). Consumer-delivered services as a best practice in mental health care delivery and the development of practice guidelines. *Psychiatric Rehabilitation Skills, 6*(3), 355–383.

Substance Abuse and Mental Health Services Administration, Office of Applied Studies (SAMHSA) (2008). *Results from the 2007 national survey on drug use and health: National findings.* NSDUH Series H-34, DHHS Publication No. SMA 08-4343. Rockville, MD.

Substance Abuse and Mental Health Services Administration, Office of Applied Studies (2008). *The DASIS report: First-time and repeat admissions aged 18–25 to substance abuse treatment 2006.* Rockville, MD.

Wechsler, H., & Weuthrich, B. (2002). *Dying to drink: Confronting binge drinking on college campuses.* New York, NY: St. Martin's Press.

White, W. L., & Finch, A. J. (2006). The recovery school movement: Its history and future. *Counselor, 7*(2), 54–57.

Willis, T. A., & Shinar, O. (2000). Measuring perceived and received social support. In S. Cohen, L. G. Underwood, & B. H. Gottlieb (Eds.), *Social support measurement and intervention* (pp. 86–135). New York: Oxford University Press.

Subject Index

Note: The letters 'f' and 't' following the locators refer to figures and tables respectively.

H.H. Cleveland et al. (eds.), *Substance Abuse Recovery in College,* Advancing Responsible Adolescent Development, DOI 10.1007/978-1-4419-1767-6, © Springer Science+Business Media, LLC 2010